Student Workbook

SPORTS INJURY MANAGEMENT

Student Workbook

Prepared by:

Malissa Martin, Ph.D., A.T.,C.
Director, Athletic Training Curriculum Program
Department of Physical Education
University of South Carolina
Columbia, South Carolina

To Accompany the First Edition of:

SPORTS INJURY MANAGEMENT

Marcia K. Anderson, Ph.D., L.A.T.,C.
Professor and Director, Athletic Training Curriculum Program
Department of Movement Arts, Health Promotions, and Leisure Studies
Bridgewater State College
Bridgewater, Massachusetts

Susan J. Hall, Ph.D.
Professor and Director of Graduate Studies
Department of Kinesiology and Physical Education
California State University, Northridge
Northridge, California

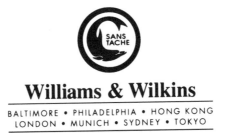

Williams & Wilkins

BALTIMORE • PHILADELPHIA • HONG KONG
LONDON • MUNICH • SYDNEY • TOKYO

A WAVERLY COMPANY

1995

Executive Editor: Donna Balado
Developmental Editor: Victoria Vaughn
Production Coordinator: Peter J. Carley
Project Editor: Arlene Sheir-Allen

Accurate indications, adverse reactions, and dosage schedules for drugs are provided in this book, but it is possible they may change. The reader is urged to review the package information data of the manufacturers of the medications mentioned.

Printed in the United States of America

The Publishers have made every effort to trace the copyright holders for borrowed material. If they have inadvertently overlooked any, they will be pleased to make the necessary arrangements at the first opportunity.

95 96 97 98 99
2 3 4 5 6 7 8 9 10

Reprints of chapters may be purchased from Williams & Wilkins in quantities of 100 or more. Call Isabella Wise, Special Sales Department, (800) 358-3583.

Preface

This Student Workbook was written specifically for the first edition of *Sports Injury Management.* The purpose of the workbook is to provide the student with useful exercises and experiences to reinforce and enhance the concepts and material presented in the text. The workbook provides the student with an active learning, problem solving and critical thinking approach to situations involved in athletic training and athletic health care.

Designed to correspond with the chapters of the text, chapters in this workbook include:

Learning Objectives...pinpoints important student learning goals

Anatomy Review...provides for a review of anatomical structures associated with the chapter

Key Terminology...stresses important terms and their meaning

Kinematics...provides for range of motion, muscle action, and functional measurements

Simulations...provides for critical thinking exercises through the use of injury scenarios, leading the student from one part of the scenario to the next. Many of the scenarios parallel those presented in the text and Instructor's Manual

Situations...provides for critical thinking exercises associated with specific athletic injury situations

Special Tests...stresses the special tests used in the evaluation of specific athletic injuries

Multiple Choice Questions...

Additional Activities...provides for additional learning activities to be used as educational enhancing experiences for the student

A special thanks to: Marcia Anderson for asking me to develop and write the student workbook for *Sports Injury Management* and giving me an opportunity for another learning experience; Andy Bosman for his expertise, time, and patience in doing the desktop publishing for the workbook; Kim Shibinski, who has given me the support and encouragement to continue to reach for my dreams and accomplish my goals; and the 1994 to 1995 senior and junior athletic training students in the University of South Carolina program for giving me the opportunity to work through each chapter with them prior to publication. Their efforts and dedication will always be appreciated.

Malissa Martin

CONTENTS

Chapter 1

Sports Injury Management and the Athletic Trainer

After completing this chapter you should be able to:

- Identify health care services in sports medicine that enhance health fitness and sport performance.

- Identify members of the primary sports medicine team, their role and responsibility in sport injury management.

- Explain basic parameters of ethical conduct and standards of professional practice for athletic trainers.

- Specify academic and clinical requirements necessary to become a National Athletic Trainers' Association (NATA) certified athletic trainer, and continuing education requirements needed to maintain certification.

- Explain standard of care of what factors must be proved to show breach of duty of care.

- Describe preventative measures to reduce potential risk of litigation.

- Discuss potential job opportunities for an individual interested in athletic training as a career option.

I. Key Terms

Instructions: *On a separate sheet of paper define the following terms.*

Sports medicine	Tort	Nonfeasance
Standard of care	Battery	Malpractice
Informed consent	Foreseeability of harm	Implied warranty
Negligence	Malfeasance	Expressed warranty
Gross negligence	Misfeasance	Modalities

II. Simulations

Instructions: *Perform the following simulated experiences.*

You have learned that several high school athletes are using the weight room when a supervisor is not present. Although the athletes have been instructed in proper lifting technique and safety, you are concerned about legal liability. What implications exist concerning your legal responsibility to these athletes?

1A. What actions should be taken to ensure a safe weight room facility?

You are a college athletic trainer and you have a student who wants to pursue NATA certification. There is no accredited curriculum program at your college. How will you guide and help this student in his/her pursuit?

2A. You have successfully passed the NATA certification examination, and you are now a certified athletic trainer. What type of continuing education requirements must you know?

III. Situations

Instructions: *Work with a partner to cooperatively analyze and answer the following situations.*

1. You have just been named the athletic trainer at a major high school. You are the first athletic trainer in the history of the high school and must develop a sports medicine team. What individuals might you have on your team?

2. You are a high school athletic trainer and have just been asked by your athletic director to justify your position at the school to the school board. How would you do this?

3. An athlete sustains an injury. What standards of care and professional conduct should the athlete expect from an immediate health care provider?

III. Situations (Con't)

4. A soccer player received a severe blow to the anterior right thigh that resulted in rapid swelling. The athletic trainer applied ice to limit swelling and referred the athlete to a physician. The athlete decided not to see the physician and returned home to ice the leg. Three days later the swelling was still present, and the soccer player had problems moving the foot of the injured leg. If litigation occurred as a result of this injury, what should the athletic trainer have done to protect against possible legal action?

IV. Multiple Choice Questions

Instructions: *Choose the best answer for each question.*

____1. The first primary duty of an athletic trainer is:
    a. injury rehabilitation   c. education and counseling
    b. injury prevention   d. administration of preseason physical

____2. Injury management follows what duty of the athletic trainer?
    a. injury prevention   c. dispensing of medications
    b. review of preseason physical   d. recognition and injury evaluation

____3. In the absence of an athletic trainer, the _____must assume a more active role in providing health care to sport participants.
    a. coach   c. student athletic trainer
    b. faculty member   d. equipment manager

____4. Students who attend an accredited athletic training curriculum program must complete ____clinical hours under the supervision of a NATA certified athletic trainer.
    a. 1500   c. 1000
    b. 800   d. 1200

____5. _____ and _____ are two of the strongest safeguards against litigation for athletic trainers.
    a. being properly licensed and practicing within established standards of practice
    b. being nationally certified and having full-time employment
    c. being properly licensed and having current first-aid and CPR certification
    d. being nationally certified and having liability insurance coverage

____6. The final authority to clear an athlete for participation rests with the:
    a. athletic trainer   c. supervising physician
    b. coach   d. school nurse

____7. An athletic trainer suspects a football player has a neck injury but does not use a rigid backboard to stabilize the individual. What type of legal liability could result from the athletic trainer's actions?
    a. malfeasance   c. gross negligence
    b. nonfeasance   d. malpractice

_____8. While on a road trip, an athletic trainer dispenses prescription medication to an athlete who is suffering from a cold. What type of legal liability could result from the athletic trainer's actions?

a. malfeasance
b. failure to warn
c. nonfeasance
d. misfeasance

_____9. Failure to receive informed consent from an athlete could result in:

a. gross negligence
b. misfeasance
c. battery
d. tort

_____10. _____has established minimum standards for football helmets and their use.

a. OSHA
b. NOCSAE
c. NCAA
d. NAIA

_____11. The statute of limitation for accident reports range from __ to ___, depending upon state law.

a. 6 to 12 months
b. 1 to 3 years
c. 1 to 5 years
d. 3 to 7 years

_____12. While taking an athlete's medical history, it has been noted that the athlete has only one kidney. What type of sport is recommended that this athlete not participate in?

a. noncontact strenuous
b. limited contact/collision
c. contact/collision
d. noncontact/nonstrenuous

_____13. Traditional athletic training settings are considered to be in:

a. sports medicine clinics
b. industrial clinics
c. college and high schools
d. colleges only

_____14. An athlete is down on the field with a possible head/neck injury. An athletic trainer, team physician, neurologist, and EMT are on the field caring for the injured athlete. Who should be in charge of moving and transporting the injured athlete?

a. neurologist
b. EMT
c. team physician
d. athletic trainer

_____15. While participating in an away contest, an athlete sustains an injury that needs transportation to a medical facility. What type of record should be available to determine if the athlete has allergies to medications?

a. medical data information card
b. physical examination record
c. accident report
d. daily injury report

V. Additional Activities

1. **Develop a preseason physical for a team or group of athletes. In your plan include forms, needed personnel, equipment, examination stations, and procedures.**

2. **Develop forms used for record-keeping procedures in athletic training.**

3. **Design a sports medicine team indicating roles and duties of each member.**

4. **Develop a policy and procedure manual for an athletic training program.**

I. Key Terms

Sports medicine — — — — Area of health and special services that apply medical and scientific knowledge to prevent, recognize, manage, and rehabilitate injuries related to sport, exercise, and/or recreational activity.

Standard of care — — — — What action another minimally competent professional educated and practicing in the same profession would have taken in the same or similar circumstance to protect an individual from harm.

Informed consent — — — Condition whereby an injured adult, or parents of minor children, has been reasonably informed of needed treatment, possible alternative treatments, and advantages and disadvantages of each course of action, and gives written consent to receive treatment.

Negligence — — — — — Breach of one's duty of care that causes harm to another individual.

Gross negligence — — — Breach of one's duty of care that causes harm to another individual.

Tort — — — — — — — A wrong done to an individual whereby the injured party seeks a remedy for damages suffered.

Battery — — — — — — Unpermitted or intentional contact with another individual without their consent.

Foreseeability of harm — — Condition whereby danger is apparent, or should have be apparent, resulting in an unreasonably unsafe condition.

Malfeasance — — — — — Committing an act that is not your responsibility to perform.

Misfeasance — — — — — Committing an act that is your responsibility to perform, but the wrong procedure is followed, or the right procedure is done in an improper manner.

Nonfeasance — — — — — Failing to perform one's legal duty of care.

Malpractice — — — — — Committing a negligent act while providing care.

Implied warranty — — — Unwritten guarantee that the product is reasonably safe when used for its intended purpose.

Expressed warranty — — Written guarantee that states the product is safe for consumer use.

Modalities — — — — — — Therapeutic agents that enhance tissue healing while reducing pain and disability.

II. Simulations

 Legal Liability

Did you determine what your duty of care is relative to the athletes lifting weights in an unsupervised weight room? Did you take the following course of action:
- foresee the possibility of injury
- warn the individuals to leave the weight room
- take immediate action to close the weight room until competent personnel could supervise the area.

Failure to perform these actions could make the athletic trainer liable through the act of nonfeasance.

1A. Did your preventive measures include:
- posting signs that no one is allowed in the weight room unless supervised by competent personnel
- posting signs on the walls of the weight room depicting proper lifting techniques for each lift
- locking the weight room when there is no supervisor

Did you determine that the following need to be accomplished prior to the individual becoming a certified athletic trainer?
- the completion of formal instruction in anatomy/physiology, kinesiology/biomechanics, exercise physiology, basic athletic training, and advanced athletic training.
- 1500 clinical hours under the direct supervision of a certified athletic trainer
- proof of graduation at the baccalaureate level at an accredited college or university
- at least 25% of clinical athletic training experiences must be attained in practice and/or game coverage with one or more of the following sports: football, soccer, wrestling, gymnastics, hockey, wrestling, basketball, lacrosse, volleyball, and rugby
- endorsement by a certified athletic trainer
- current CPR certification
- success in passing the NATA examination

2A.Did you determine that after an individual becomes certified that individual must meet the following continuing education requirements to maintain certification?
- eight continuing education units over a three-year period
- current proof of CPR certification at least once during the three-year period

Refer to pages 13–14 in the text.

III. Situations

1. **Sports Medicine Team** - Did your sports medicine team include:
    - team physician
    - athletic trainer
    - primary care physician
    - other professional health personnel

    Refer to Table 1-1 on page 6 in the text.

2. **Duties of the athletic trainer** - Did you include the following duties to justify your position as an athletic trainer?
    - injury prevention
    - recognition and evaluation of injuries/illnesses
    - injury management/treatment and disposition
    - injury rehabilitation
    - organization and administration of athletic health care
    - education and counseling of athletes

    Refer to Table 1-2 on page 9 in text.

III. Situations (Con't)

3. Standard of Professional Practice - Did you determine that the individual providing the care should be an NATA certified athletic trainer and that the standard of care should reflect the profession of athletic training?

4. Injury report - In administering care to the injured soccer player, did you determine that an injury report should be completed documenting the injury and the need to see a physician?

Refer to Field Strategy 1-7 on page 28 in the text.

IV. Multiple Choice Answers

1. b	6. c	11. d
2. d	7. b	12. c
3. a	8. a	13. c
4. b	9. c	14. b
5. a	10. b	15. a

2 The Mechanics of Tissue Injury and Healing

After completing this chapter you should be able to:

- Define compression, tension, shear, stress, strain, bending, and torsion and explain how each can play a role in injury to biological tissue

- Explain how the material constituent and structural organization of skin, tendon, ligament, muscle, and bone affect the ability of these structures to withstand the mechanical loads to which each is subjected

- List and describe common injuries of skin, tendons, ligaments, muscles, and bone

- Describe the processes by which nerves are injured and the processes by which nerves can heal

- Discuss the types of altered sensation that can result from nerve injury

I. Key Terms

Instructions: *On a separate sheet of paper define the following terms.*

Torsion	Adhesions	Tendinitis
Bending	Stress	Tenosynovitis
Yield point	Osteopenia	Calcific tendinitis
Anisotropic	Failure	Bursitis
Viscoelastic	Fracture	Fascitis
Zone of primary injury	Stress fracture	Hypoxia
Zone of secondary injury	Callus	Necrosis
Cancellous	Cramp	Dermatome
Cortical	Spasm	Afferent nerves
Chemosensitive	Contusion	Efferent nerves
Mechanosensitive	Myositis	Nociceptors
Phagocytosis	Myositis ossificans	Neuroma
Edema	Hematoma	Neurotmesis
Ecchymosis	Strain	Amenorrhea

II. Simulations

Instructions: *Perform the following simulated experiences.*

 A runner reports to you with localized shin pain that has been increasingly bothersome for a few weeks. What type of injury/injuries might you suspect?

1A. Since the runner's pain has been present for a few weeks, it probably is a chronic or stress injury. In reference to the runner's training, what suggestions can you give to reduce the incidence of this injury recurring?

 A baseball player was hit in the thigh by a wild pitch while batting. What injuries should be suspected? If the injury is superficial, what signs and symptoms might you suspect?

2A. After noting the signs and symptoms associated with a superficial contusion, demonstrate how to determine the severity of this injury.

 A weight lifter complains of pain radiating down the posterior aspect of the leg along with hypesthesia. What condition might you suspect and why?

3A. Knowing that radiating pain and hypesthesia might indicate nerve involvement, describe the treatment protocol for this injury?

III. Situations

Instructions: *Work with a partner to cooperatively analyze and answer the following situations.*

l. A running back was sandwiched between two players while being tackled. As a result, the running back sustained a thigh contusion. What type of load and force was associated with this injury?

2. A rugby player's leg is anchored to the ground and is tackled on that leg from the front while being pushed into the tackle from behind. A bending moment is created on the lower leg. What type of injury do you suspect to occur to the lower leg?

III. Situations (Con't)

3. An athlete approaches you and questions why he/she has been told to do static stretching for a period of 30 seconds for each stretch rather than doing short ballistic stretches. How would you address this question?

4. A basketball player has sustained an ankle injury. Describe degrees of injury including crepitus, tissue damage, and signs and symptoms.

5. An athlete reports to you complaining of pain over the big toe. The athlete reports no recollection of injury. How would you determine if the toe is inflamed?

6. An adolescent athlete has sustained a routine ankle sprain. The pain continues to be localized at the joint line. After 2 weeks of conservative treatment, there is little to no improvement in the signs or symptoms of the injury. What type of injury should be suspected and why?

7. A sedentary 60-year-old woman wants to begin a weight-bearing exercise program. What precautions should be taken to prevent a bone injury? Why?

IV. Multiple Choice Questions

Instructions: *Choose the best answer for each question.*

___1. When a force is sustained by the tissues of the human body, two primary factors help determine whether injury results. These primary factors are:
a. the size of the tissue and magnitude of the force
b. the magnitude of the force and the material properties of the tissue
c. the acceleration and target of the force
d. the mechanical load and compression of the force

___2. When a load exceeds a material's yield point, the response of the material is:
a. elastic   c. plastic
b. deformation   d. anisotropic

___3. Axial loading that produces a crushing effect is termed _____. This occurs when a football player is sandwiched between two opposing players.
a. deformation   c. compression
b. tensile force   d. shearing force

___4. Spondylolisthesis, a condition involving anterior slippage of a vertebra with respect to the vertebra below it, is often due to a _____type of force.
a. compression   c. tensile
b. decompression   d. shearing

___5. The amount of torque produced in a body part is the product of ____ with respect to the joint center.
   a. muscle acceleration and the muscle's moment arm
   b. muscle force and the muscle's moment arm
   c. shearing forces and forced acceleration
   d. compression and magnitude of force

___6. Bones will normally resist _____ forces better than tension forces.
   a. compression   c. chronic
   b. acute   d. shearing

___7. Because of a muscle's ____, a static stretch maintained for 30 seconds is more effective than a series of short ballistic stretches.
   a. extensibility   c. viscoelastic aspects
   b. contractility   d. irritability

___8. A muscle will only shorten when the tension developed by that muscle is:
   a. isometric   c. eccentric
   b. concentric   d. elastic

___9. Abrasions and blisters are a result of ____ force.
   a. shear   c. compression
   b. tension   d. tensile

___10. After sustaining a contusion to the right thigh, the athlete notices a hard mass that is causing pain and some paralysis in his leg. What might be developing in this athlete's leg?
   a. bruise   c. hematoma
   b. muscle spasm   d. myositis

___11. A tendon or ligament injury that demonstrates severe pain, extensive rupturing of tissue, detectable joint instability, and/or muscle weakness is indicative of a:
   a. first degree sprain or strain   c. third degree sprain or strain
   b. second degree sprain or strain d. mild injury

___12. Bursitis may be acute or chronic and may be caused by a single traumatic ____or repeated ____associated with overuse of the joint.
   a. tensile force, compression   c. compression, shearing force
   b. shearing force, tension   d. compression, compression

___13. The beginning of the acute phase of injury involves ____, lasting from a few seconds to as long as 10 minutes.
   a. vasodilation   c. spasms
   b. vasoconstriction   d. necrosis

___14. Platelets and basophil leukocytes transport histamine to the injury site that serves as a _____ and increases blood vessel permeability.
   a. vasodilator   c. vasoconstrictor
   b. leukocyte   d. hypoxic

___15. Applying ice, compression and elevation to an acute injury decreases injury to the ____.
   a. zone of primary injury   c. zone of secondary injury
   b. soft tissue   d. associated bone

___16. Because scar tissue is_____, it can reduce a structure's tensile strength by as much as ___percent as compared to preinjury strength.

a. elastic, 30   c. elastic, 50

b. inelastic, 30   d. inelastic, 50

___17. The amount of atrophy in a structure is proportional to the time of:

a. mobilization of the structure   c. immoblization of the structure

b. injury   d. year the injury occurs

___18. Pinching the sciatic nerve at its root may cause pain along the nerve's course down the posterior aspect of the leg. This type of pain is known as:

a. referred pain   c. intermittent

b. radiating   d. delayed

___19. During adolescence, ligaments and tendons tend to be stronger than bone. This makes the adolescent athlete at higher risk for ____fractures.

a. greenstick   c. avulsion

b. spiral   d. oblique

___20. Apophysitis, seen in adolescents and children, is often associated with traumatic ___type fractures.

a. avulsion   c. epiphyseal

b. impacted   d. stress

V. Additional Activities

1. Describe how forces affect the mechanism of injury.

2. Explain the various injuries to both soft and hard tissue.

3. List the types of epiphyseal injuries, and explain the differences between the immature and mature musculoskeletal system.

4. Using a diagrammatic representation, explain the process of soft tissue healing.

I. Key Terms

Torsion — — — — — — — Twisting around an object's longitudinal axis in response to an applied torque

Bending — — — — — — — Loading that produces tension on one side of an object and compression on the other side

Yield point — — — — — The maximum load that a material can sustain without permanent deformation

Anisotropic — — — — — Having different strengths in response to loads from different directions

Viscoelastic — — — — — Responding to loading over time with changing rates of deformation

Zone of primary injury —— Region of injured tissue prior to vasodilation

Zone of secondary injury — Region of damaged tissue following vasodilation

Cancellous — — — — — Bone tissue of relatively low density

Cortical — — — — — — Compact bone tissue of relatively high density

Chemosensitive — — — — Sensitive to chemical stimulation

Mechanosensitive — — — Sensitive to mechanical stimulation

Phagocytosis — — — — — Process by which white blood cells surround and digest foreign particles

Edema — — — — — — — Swelling resulting from collection of exuded lymph fluid in the interstitial tissues

Ecchymosis — — — — — Superficial tissue discoloration

Adhesions — — — — — — Tissues that bind the healing tissue to adjacent structures, such as other ligaments or bone

Stress — — — — — — — The distribution of force within a body; quantified as force divided by the area over which the force acts

I. Key Terms (Con't)

Osteopenia — — — — — Condition of reduced bone mineral density that predisposes the individual to fractures

Failure — — — — — — Loss of continuity; rupture of soft tissue or fracture of the bone

Fracture — — — — — — A disruption in the continuity of a bone

Stress fracture — — — — — Fracture resulting from repeated loading with relatively low magnitude of force

Callus — — — — — — — Fibrous tissue containing immature bone tissue that forms at fracture sites during repair and regeneration

Cramp — — — — — — Painful involuntary muscle contraction, either clonic or tonic

Spasm — — — — — — — Transitory muscle contractions

Contusion — — — — — — Compression injury involving accumulation of blood and lymph within a muscle

Myositis — — — — — — Inflammation of connective tissue within a muscle

Myositis ossificans — — — Accumulation of mineral deposits in a muscle

Hematoma — — — — — — A localized mass of blood and lymph confined within a space or tissue

Strain — — — — — — — Amount of deformation with respect to the original dimensions of the structure

Tendinitis — — — — — — Inflammation of a tendon

Tenosynovitis — — — — — Inflammation of a tendon sheath

Calcific tendinitis — — — Accumulation of mineral deposits in a tendon

Bursitis — — — — — — Inflammation of a bursa

Fascitis — — — — — — Inflammation of the fascia surrounding portions of a muscle

Hypoxia — — — — — — Having a reduced concentration of oxygen

Necrosis — — — — — — Death of a tissue

Key Terms (Con't)

Dermatome — — — — — A region of the skin supplied by a single afferent neuron

Afferent nerves — — — — Nerves carrying sensory input from receptors in the skin, muscles, tendons, and ligaments to the central nervous system

Efferent nerves — — — — Nerves carrying stimuli from the central nervous system to the muscles

Nociceptors — — — — — Specialized nerve endings that transduce pain

Neuroma — — — — — — A nerve tumor

Neurotmesis — — — — — Complete severance of a nerve

Amenorrhea — — — — — Condition involving cessation of menses

II. Simulations

1 Chronic Injury

Did you suspect the runner's injury was a chronic or stress injury?

1A. To decrease the recurrence of this injury, did you suggest progression of intensity, change in running surface, and change in shoes during conditioning sessions?

2 Superficial Contusion

Did you suspect the baseball player had a contusion? Did you note that ecchymosis may be present if the hemorrhage is superficial?

2A. To determine the severity of the contusion, did you have the injured athlete perform knee range of motion to note limitations in movement?

3 Nerve Injury

Because of the radiating pain, did you identify that the weight lifter may be experiencing some sort of nerve injury?

3A. Did your treatment plan include medical referral?

III. Situations

l. Axial Load - Did you determine that an axial load and compression force were associated with the thigh contusion of the running back?

2. Lower Leg Fracture - Did you determine what may have occurred when a tension force was applied to the leg of the rugby player? Since a bone can resist compression forces much better than tension forces, did you identify that a possible fracture may have occurred?

3. Stretching - Did you determine that because of the viscoelastic aspect of muscle extensibility, it enables the muscle to stretch to greater lengths over time in response to a sustained tensile force. A static stretch maintained over a period of 30 seconds is more effective in increasing muscle length than a series of short ballistic stretches.

4. Ankle Injury - Did you look for the following signs and symptoms to determine the degree of injury to the basketball player's ankle?
    -degree of discomfort and pain
    -local tenderness
    -degree of swelling
    -ecchymosis
    -function

5. Inflammation - Did you determine that inflammation of the big toe would exhibit the following signs and symptoms?
    -redness (rubor)
    -local heat (calor)
    -swelling (tumor)
    -pain (dolor)
    -loss of function (function laesa)

6. Epiphyseal Injury - Did you suspect an ankle epiphyseal injury in the adolescent athlete? Did you derive this conclusion based on the age of the athlete and the lack of improvement of the injury after conservative treatment?

7. Senior Athlete - Did you suggest that the 60-year-old woman should begin her weight-bearing exercise progressively so her bones could adapt to exercise and activity? Did you determine that this adaptation is necessary because of bone deterioration as a result of the aging process and lack of previous weight-bearing activity?

IV. Multiple Choice Answers

l. b	8. b	15. c
2. c	9. a	16. b
3. c	10. c	17. c
4. d	11. b	18. b
5. b	12. d	19. c
6. a	13. b	20. a
7. c	14. c	

Chapter 3 — Emergency Procedures

After completing this chapter you should be able to:

- Describe the signs, symptoms, and management of potentially life-threatening conditions

- Identify preventative measures to reduce the risk of life-threatening conditions

- Indicate major components of an emergency procedures plan

- Describe the procedures and techniques used in a primary and secondary injury assessment

- Identify emergency conditions that warrant immediate action by emergency medical services (EMS)

- Describe proper procedures to transport a seriously injured individual

I. Key Terms

Instructions: *On a separate sheet of paper define the following terms.*

Primary survey	Diastole	Acclimatization
Secondary survey	Systole	Hyperthermia
Triage	Cyanosis	Hypothermia
Emergency plan	Pallor	Heat cramps
Sign	Rubor	Cold urticaria
Symptom	Pupillary light reflex	Cold diuresis
Vital signs	Diplopia	Diuretics
Unconsciousness	Syncope	Raynaud's phenomenon
Partial airway obstruction	Crepitus	Hemophilia
Total airway obstruction	Decerebrate rigidity	Hemostasis
Dyspnea	Decorticate rigidity	Ad libitum
Apnea		

II. Simulations

Instructions: *Perform the following simulated experiences.*

 While participating in the Senior Games, an elderly man begins to complain of chest pains after his swimming event. What questions should be asked to determine the extent of his complaint?

1A. After questioning the senior athlete, you have determined that he may be experiencing a heart attack. How will you handle this situation?

 You have been called onto the field during a football game. After completing a primary and secondary survey, you suspect the player may have a lower leg fracture. Demonstrate the immediate first-aid procedures for this injury.

2A. After calling EMS and immobilizing the lower leg, think for a minute or two about what possible complications might occur as a result of this traumatic injury. What are these complications? How can you reduce their incidence?

 A wrestler leaves the mat during the match because of heavy and deep breathing. He is somewhat dizzy, disoriented, and is sweating profusely. What condition may be present, and what is your immediate reaction?

3A. The wrestler is experiencing heat exhaustion. What signs and symptoms would lead you to believe the condition is deteriorating into heat stroke? How can you lessen the risk of this occurring?

 A downhill skier is complaining of numbness and pain in the fingers and toes. Upon observation, you notice these areas are red and swollen, yet cold to the touch. What condition may be present? How should it be treated?

4A. What signs and symptoms would indicate the presence of deep frostbite?

5 A gymnast slipped off the springboard on an approach to a vault and collided full force into the vaulting horse. The individual is now lying on the floor motionless. What immediate care should be provided to this individual? How should additional help be summoned?

5A. In initiating the facility's emergency procedures plan, what priorities need to be assessed to determine if any life-threatening condition is present?

5B. The gymnast was not moving as you approached. As you moved closer, however, the individual groans and moves an arm. You have determined that breathing and circulation are present. The gymnast is somewhat lethargic. Breathing is shallow, but pulse is normal. Proceed to the secondary survey but continue to monitor vitals signs. What are the vital signs?

5C. The gymnast reported pain on the left side of the chest and increased pain during deep inhalations. There is discoloration present on the lower left side of the anterior chest wall. Palpation elicited pain in the region of the ninth and tenth rib on the lateral side and increased with compression on the sternum. Muscle strength and sensation in the hands and feet appear normal. Should you activate EMS?

5D. What type of information should be provided to the EMS upon arrival at the scene? Should an injury report form be completed?

III. Situations

Instructions: *Work with a partner to cooperatively analyze and answer the following situations.*

l. You are watching a field hockey game when a player stops running and suddenly grabs the throat with both hands and appears to be choking. The athlete is becoming cyanotic. How will you handle this situation?

2. You entered the locker room to find an individual lying unconscious on the floor. Think for a minute or two about what conditions may cause unconsciousness. What are they?

3. A second baseman collided with a runner and was cleated across the front of the shin. The area is bleeding profusely. How will you control bleeding and decrease the risk of infection? What guidelines will determine if the individual can reenter the game?

III. Situations (Con't)

4. After a kick toward the goal, a soccer player lands in a fire ant bed. The player gets up and continues playing; however, you notice the athlete's skin becoming red and swollen. The player is having trouble breathing and feels lethargic. What do you suspect is occurring, and how will you handle this situation?

5. You are responsible for measuring the heat stress index prior to football practice. How is this measured? What activity should be used to prevent heat illnesses? In addition to monitoring the heat stress index, what other steps can be taken to decrease the risk of heat emergencies?

6. You have been asked to speak to a group of hikers who are going backpacking in the winter. What suggestions might you provide to prevent hypothermia during the trip?

7. A football player is down on the field. Because of the mechanism of injury, you suspect a possible head or neck injury. As you arrive, you notice the player is having difficulty breathing, and you have determined it is necessary to gain access to the airway. Demonstrate how you would open the airway in this situation. What techniques or tests would you perform to determine a possible neurological injury?

IV. Special Tests

Instructions: *Perform the following special tests and explain the rational for each test.*

-**Blood pressure measurement**
-**Respiration rate measurement**
-**Response to verbal and motor commands**

-**Pulse rate measurement**
-**Pupil reaction**

V. Multiple Choice Questions

Instructions: *Choose the best answer for each question.*

___1. Blurred vision, ringing in the ears, dizziness, and fatigue are all:
    a. signs   c. symptoms
    b. emergency situations   d. chronic injuries

___2. An athlete grasps his throat and is unable to speak or cough. What do you suspect is wrong with the athlete?
    a. the athlete is in shock
    b. the athlete is choking
    c. the athlete is hemorrhaging internally
    d. the athlete is experiencing hypothermia

___3. A spectator is experiencing pain radiating down the left arm into the neck and jaw and is having shortness of breath. What may the spectator be experiencing?
a. a heart attack   c. a strained chest muscle
b. severe shock   d. hyperthermia

___4. In emergency situations, consciousness is determined by:
a. testing of reflexes   c. verbal and sensory stimuli
b. verbal stimuli and reflex testing   d. degree of shock and hemorrhage

___5. An athlete who is severely hemorrhaging will have a _____pulse.
a. rapid and strong   c. slow and strong
b. slow and weak   d. rapid and weak

___6. Spinal, abdominal, and thoracic injuries and those injuries that produce severe pain or bleeding should always be treated for:
a. shock   c. hypotension
b. hypertension   d. hyperthermia

___7. An athlete has been bitten by a fire ant. What type of shock could result from the fire ant bite?
a. metabolic   c. anaphylactic
b. psychogenic   d. hypovolemic

___8. An athlete has sustained a fractured humerus. How would you check for circulation?
a. check a proximal pulse
b. check the distal pulse
c. ask the athlete to move the fingers of the injured arm
d. check the color of the athlete's tongue

___9. As air temperature approaches body temperature and exceeds 30.6° C, _____becomes the major means of heat dissipation.
a. conduction   c. radiation
b. convection   d. evaporation

___10. _____is the most important factor that determines the effectiveness of evaporated heat loss.
a. relative humidity   c. wind speed
b. temperature   d. barometric pressure

___11. The NCAA recommends a gradual participation over _____days to provide an adequate acclimatization to the environment.
a. 1 to 3   c. 7 to 14
b. 7 to 10   d. 5

___12. Athletes who have had diarrhea should be closely watched for possible:
a. stress fractures   c. shock
b. hypertension   d. dehydration

___13. An athlete exhibits signs of disorientation, shallow breathing, hot, dry, reddish skin, and rapid, strong pulse. What do you think this athlete is experiencing?
a. heat exhaustion   c. hypothermia
b. heat stroke   d. shock

___14. Localized frostbite occurs when the core temperature _____ and the shell temperature _____.
    a. remains constant, increases   c. increases, remains constant
    b. remains constant, decreases   d. decreases, remains constant

___15. The primary survey establishes:
    a. the mechanism of injury   c. a person's responsiveness and ABCs
    b. the severity of injury   d. a person's neurological level

___16. To determine if an unconscious person is totally unresponsive, you would:
    a. shake the person
    b. call the person by name
    c. pinch the soft tissue of the person's armpit to determine if the person withdraws from stimuli
    d. check the person's pupils for responsiveness

___17. The pulse of an unconscious person should be checked at the:
    a. carotid artery   c. radial artery
    b. femoral artery   d. tibial artery

___18. The _____ of the secondary assessment helps determine the mechanism of injury.
    a. history   c. palpation
    b. observation   d. special tests

___19. ____pupils indicate possible shock, hemorrhage and cardiac arrest.
    a. constricted   c. unequal
    b. dilated   d. discolored

___20. In an emergency situation if an athlete has no response to muscular movement during special testing procedures, the athlete should be treated as having:
    a. compound fracture   c. head or neck injury
    b. heat stroke   d. internal hemorrhage

VI. Additional Activities

1. Using a sling psychrometer, determine what type of practice a team should have for a particular day.

2. Develop an emergency plan and procedure for a specific athletic facility or site.

3. Develop a plan for preventing heat illness and cold related injuries.

4. Perform a primary and secondary survey for an emergency situation.

5. Practice transporting an athlete on a stretcher by using the four or five person log roll method.

6. Attain CPR certification.

I. Key Terms

Primary survey — — — — Immediate assessment to determine unresponsiveness and status of the ABCs

Secondary survey — — — Detailed head-to-toe assessment to detect medical and injury related problems that if unrecognized and untreated could become life-threatening

Triage — — — — — — — Assessing all injured individuals to determine priority of care

Emergency plan — — — — A process that activates emergency health care services of the facility and community

Sign — — — — — — — Objective measurable physical finding that you hear, feel, see, or smell during the assessment

Symptom — — — — — Subjective information provided by an individual regarding their perception of the problem

Vital signs — — — — — Objective measurements of pulse, respirations, blood pressure, and skin temperature indicating normal body function

Unconsciousness — — — — Impairment of brain function whereby the individual lacks conscious awareness and is unable to respond to superficial sensory stimuli

Partial airway obstruction — Choking where the individual has some air exchange in the lungs and is able to cough

Total airway obstruction — Choking where the individual has no air passing through vocal cords and is unable to speak or cough

Dyspnea — — — — — — Labored or difficult breathing

Apnea — — — — — — — Temporary cessation of breathing

Diastole — — — — — — Residual pressure in the aorta between heart beats

Systole — — — — — — Pressure in the aorta when the left ventricle contracts

I. Key Terms (Con't)

Cyanosis — — — — — — — A dark bluish or purple tinge to the skin due to deficient oxygen in the blood

Pallor — — — — — — — Skin ashen or pale in color

Rubor — — — — — — — Skin reddish in color

Pupillary light reflex — — Rapid constriction of pupils when exposed to intense light

Diplopia — — — — — — Double vision

Syncope — — — — — — Fainting or light-headedness

Crepitus — — — — — — Cracking or grating sound heard during palpation that indicates a possible fracture

Decerebrate rigidity — — — Extension of all four extremities

Decorticate rigidity — — — Extension of the legs with flexion of the elbows, wrists, and fingers

Acclimatization — — — — Physiologic adaptations of an individual to a different environment, especially climate or altitude

Hyperthermia — — — — — Elevated body temperature

Hypothermia — — — — — Decreased body temperature

Heat cramps — — — — — Painful involuntary muscle spasms caused by excessive water and electrolyte loss

Cold urticaria — — — — — Condition characterized by redness, itching, and large blister-like wheals on skin that is exposed to cold

Cold diuresis — — — — — Excretion of urine in cold weather due to blood being shunted away from the skin to the core to maintain vascular volume

Diuretics — — — — — — Drugs that promote the excretion of urine

Raynaud's phenomenon — Condition characterized by intermittent bilateral attacks of ischemia of the fingers or toes, marked by severe pallor, numbness, and pain

Hemophilia — — — — — — Inability of blood to clot, which can lead to excessive blood loss

Hemostasis — — — — — — The state of equilibrium within the body's various tissues and systems

Ad libitum — — — — — — At pleasure or at will

II. Simulations

 Heart Attack Victim

Did your questions include:
- pain originating behind the sternum and radiating into either or both arms, neck, jaws, teeth, or upper back
- shortness of breath, nausea, and a feeling of impending doom
- past history of heart problems

1A. Did you determine that the senior athlete may be experiencing a heart attack and summon EMS immediately?

2 **Lower Leg Fracture**

Did the immediate first-aid procedures for the football player's lower leg fracture include:
- checking for a distal pulse and cutaneous sensation
- immobilizing the lower leg with a splint above the knee and below the ankle
- elevating the lower leg after immobilization
- monitoring vital signs
- activating EMS or transporting to a physician

2A. Did you determine that a complication from a fracture may be shock and therefore should be treated for shock?

3 **Heat Emergencies**

Refer to Field Strategy 3-5 on page 75 in the text.

Did you suspect that the wrestler was experiencing heat exhaustion? Did the treatment plan include:
    -moving the wrestler to a cool place
    -removing equipment and unnecessary clothing
    -administering cool fluids
    -elevating the wrestler's feet above heart level
    -monitoring vital signs
    -activating EMS

3A. Did you note the following signs and symptoms that would indicate the wrestler's condition was deteriorating into heat stroke?
    -increased temperature
    -hot and dry skin
    -lack of sweating
    -rapid, strong pulse
    -dilated pupils
    -unconsciousness

4 **Frostbite**

Refer to Table 3-7 on page 78 in the text.

Did you suspect the skier had superficial frostbite? Did your treatment include:
    - removing the person to a warm indoor location
    - carefully warm the fingers and toes rapidly by immersing them into water heated to 104 to 108° F for 30 to 45 minutes
    - when area is rewarmed, gently dry and apply sterile dressing between and over the digits
    -cover the affected area with towels or blankets to keep the area warm
    -transport the individual to medical facility

4A. Did you determine that the following signs might indicate the skier had deep frostbite?
    -skin appears blotchy white to yellow-gray or blue-gray
    -skin is hard and totally numb

(Refer to Table 3-10 on page 87 in the text; Table 3-ll on page 89 in the text; Table 3-12 on page 96 in the text, and Field Strategy 3-7 on page 80 in the text; Field Strategy 3-9 on page 86 in the text; Field Strategy 3-10 on page 90 in the text; and Field Strategy 3-ll on page 92 in the text.)

As the first person on the scene, did you initiate the facility's emergency procedure plan, perform a primary survey, summon help from colleagues, and call the local EMS?

5A. Did you perform the following steps in the primary survey to establish the level of responsiveness, breathing, and circulation in the gymnast?
- observe the individual moving or talking..call the individual by name. If the athlete is unconscious, summon EMS.
- assume a head and neck injury is presented, and if the athlete is unconscious, stabilize the head and neck
- check circulation by taking a pulse, and check breathing by watching the chest rise and fall. If the athlete does not have a pulse and is not breathing, summon EMS and begin CPR. If the athlete has a pulse but is not breathing, summon EMS and begin rescue breathing.
- observe posture and signs of deformities or other trauma
- observe skin color

5B. During the secondary survey, did you include:
- history of the injury (what, where, when, how questions)
- observe and inspect for bleeding, discoloration, swelling, deformities, skin color, pupil size, and reaction
- palpate for temperature, swelling, point tenderness, crepitus, deformity, muscle spasm, cutaneous sensation, and pulse
- special tests in muscular movements and blood pressure

Did you monitor the following vital signs?
- consciousness
- pulse and breathing rate for 30 seconds
- blood pressure
- recheck the vital signs every 3 to 5 minutes

5C. Yes, since the gymnast is having painful, limited respirations, palpable pain, and discoloration in the thoracic region, EMS should be activated to transport the gymnast to the nearest trauma center.

5D. Did you determine that the following information should be given to the EMS?
- mechanism of injury
- characteristics and duration of the symptoms and vital signs
- any muscular weakness
- changes in sensation
- treatment completed on the individual

Did you determine that an injury report form should be completed on the gymnast?

III. Situations

l. Choking Victim - Did you determine that the field hockey player was giving the universal distress sign for choking? Since the player was becoming cyanotic, did you determine that a total airway obstruction was present? You should first ask the athlete if he or she is choking. If the athlete's response is yes you should perform the Heimlich maneuver.
(Refer to text pages 82 and 83 for instructions on how to perform the Heimlich maneuver.)

2. Unconsciousness - Did you determine that the following conditions may cause unconsciousness?
- respiratory distress
- hemorrhage
- seizures or epilepsy
- heatstroke
- hypoglycemia
- drug overdose
- cerebrovascular or cardiac malfunctions
- head trauma

3. Bleeding Victim - (Refer to Field Strategy 3-l on page 62 in the text) - Did you control bleeding by first putting on latex gloves and then applying direct pressure with a sterile gauze pad to the shin? When bleeding has stopped, the wound should be cleansed with a saline solution and covered with a sterile dressing. Gloves and gauze pads containing blood should be placed in a biohazard bag. The baseball player should be referred to a physician if stitches are required.

4. Anaphylactic Shock - (Refer to Field Strategy 3-3 on page 65 in the text) - Did you suspect the soccer player was experiencing anaphylactic shock as a result of an allergic reaction to the fire ants? Did you:
- place ice on the area to reduce the inflammation
- activate EMS
- maintain an open airway
- monitor vital signs
- treat for shock

5. Heat Stress Index - (Refer to Table 3-2 on page 70 in the text) - Did you use a sling psychrometer to determine the heat stress index? Were the following wet bulb temperature range guidelines used to determine the extent of football practice:

Degrees in F	Recommendations
60	No prevention necessary
61–65	Alert athletes to symptoms of heat stress and the importance of adequate hydration
66–70	Insist that adequate water be ingested
71–75	Rest periods and water breaks every 20–30 minutes; place limits on intense activity
76–79	Modify practice considerably and curtail activity for unacclimatized athletes
80	Cancel practice

Were the following factors mentioned to decrease the risk of heat emergencies to the football team?
- identify individuals at risk
- acclimate gradually to the environment
- wear lightweight, light colored, and porous clothing
- provide adequate fluid hydration and electrolyte replacement
- utilize weight charts daily

6. Hypothermia Prevention - (Refer to Field Strategy 3-6 on page 77 in the text) - Did you suggest the following steps to prevent hypothermia?
- layer clothing
- wear clothing that includes wool, wool/synthetic blends, polypropylene, or treated polyesters such as Capilene
- wear clothing that are wind resistant such as Gortex or nylon
- wear ski-type cap, face mask, and neck warmer
- wear polypropylene gloves or woolen mittens
- wear shoes large enough to accommodate an inner layer of polypropylene socks and an outer layer of heavy wool socks
- avoid getting wet

III. Situations (Con't)

7. Football Helmet Removal - Did you determine that the football helmet should not be removed but, rather, only the face mask should be removed? To remove the facemask you should:
- stabilize the head and neck by placing the index fingers or thumbs in the helmet ear holes and hold tightly
- with the head and neck stabilized, use a screwdriver, wire cutters, or specialized tool to remove the plastic clips on the face mask
- remove the entire face mask and mouthguard to allow easy access to the mouth and nose

IV. Special Tests

Blood pressure measurement - Refer to Figure 3-22 on text page 95
Respiration rate measurement - Refer to pages 89–90 in the text
Response to verbal and motor commands - Refer to page 94 in the text
Pulse rate measurement - Refer to page 83 in the text
Pupil reaction - Refer to page 91 in the text
Also refer to Table 3-11 on page 89 in the text for information on abnormal vital signs and what they may indicate

V. Multiple Choice Answers

1. c	8. b	15. c
2. b	9. d	16. c
3. a	10. a	17. a
4. c	11. b	18. a
5. d	12. d	19. b
6. a	13. b	20. c
7. c	14. b	

Chapter 4 — Sports Injury Assessment

After completing this chapter you should be able to:

- Identify the two main body segments and demonstrate anatomical position

- Define terms relative to the direction, regions, and joint motion

- Describe HOPS injury assessment process

- Define common assessment terms

- Identify specific components in a history of an injury

- Describe what is involved in observation and inspection of an injury site

- Identify principles and techniques used in palpation, range of motion testing, neurologic testing, and special testing

- Differentiate between injury recognition and diagnosis

- Describe the components of SOAP notes and identify information recorded in each section

I. Key Terms

Instructions: *On a separate sheet of paper define the following terms.*

Etiology	Anesthesia	Closed packed position
Pathology	Hypesthesia	Loose packed position
Observation	Paresthesia	Appendicular segment
Inspection	Paresis	Axial segment
Syndrome	Referred pain	Antalgic gait
Atrophy	Somatic pain	Indication
Hypertrophy	Visceral pain	Contraindication
Ecchymosis	Goniometer	Modalities
Effusion	End feel	Diagnosis
Dermatome	Anatomical position	Prognosis
Myotome	Active movement	Sequela
Nerve root	Passive movement	Painful arc
Proprioceptors	Accessory movement	Valgus
Muscle spindle	Static position	Varus

Instructions: *Perform the following simulated experiences.*

A middle-aged tennis player is complaining of a dull, aching pain on the lateral side of the elbow. It is particularly bothersome after activity has stopped. What subjective information should be gathered to help develop a history of this injury?

1A. A history has determined that the tennis player is 52 years old and is a recreational player who plays two to three matches per week. The primary complaint is a dull, aching pain on the outside of the right elbow after completing a match. Pain is rated as a 7 on a 10- point scale and 8 when an object has to lifted. Pain persists 2 hours after play has ceased. This time is reduced when ice is applied to the elbow. There is no recollection of injury but pain has been present for the past 3 months. A physician has never been consulted about the injury. Continue assessment of the injury by performing observation and inspection procedures.

1B. During observation and inspection, the tennis player was able to perform all gross motor movements and had good posture and a normal gait. Visual inspection showed only slight redness and swelling on the lateral side of the elbow. Perform palpation.

1C. Palpation revealed warmth and slight swelling over the lateral elbow. Point tenderness was elicited directly over the lateral epicondyle of the humerus and in the soft muscle mass on the proximal forearm. All fracture tests were negative. Perform special tests.

1D. The tennis player complained of dull, aching pain on the lateral aspect of the elbow that increased after activity stopped. The painful site was isolated, and all stress tests were negative, except resisted wrist extension. This muscular movement was weak and painful. What does this positive test indicate? Does the tennis player need to see a physician?

1E. After rehabilitating the elbow of the tennis player, it is time to perform functional testing. Demonstrate functional progression for this injury.

A volleyball player reports to practice with low back pain that has been bothersome for the past 2 weeks. Perform a scan examination on this individual.

2A. The scan examination reveals limitations in trunk rotation and pain during a straight leg raise. Continue the assessment with an examination of the volleyball player's posture.

III. Situations

Instructions: *Work with a partner to cooperatively analyze and answer the following situations.*

1. A soccer player fell on an outstretched arm. You suspect a fracture above the elbow and have called the school nurse who wants to know the exact location of pain. How will you present this information so that the nurse can visualize the location of the injury and can assist you in taking the appropriate action?

2. A runner comes to you complaining of anterior hip pain. You would like to observe the individual standing in an anatomical position. How would you explain anatomical position?

3. A golfer reports to the clinic with wrist pain. What questions can be asked to determine the type and intensity of pain?

4. During a 10k road race, a runner collapses. When you arrive at the scene, the runner is conscious. Since you do not know the medical history of the runner, what questions can be asked to gather a related medical history?

5. A football player sustained a shoulder dislocation. How will you determine if the injury damaged any arteries or nerves in the area?

6. A sport participant is recovering from elbow surgery, and you need to determine elbow range of motion. Demonstrate how you would measure elbow range of motion through both subjective and objective means.

7. After performing resisted manual muscle testing following a neck injury, you have found that the player has no pain during testing but is experiencing muscle weakness. From this test, what can you conclude about the injury? Should the individual be referred to a physician for further evaluation?

8. A rugby player has sustained injury to the low back area. You are asked to determine possible central nervous system damage through the use of reflex testing. What are the various reflexes and what segmental levels are tested?

9. You work at a clinic with several employees. Why is it so important for each employee to be consistent and thorough in all injury assessments and keep accurate records? Provide an example of record keeping most often used in a sports medicine/physical therapy setting.

IV. Special Tests ———————————————————

Instructions: *Work with a partner to perform the following special tests at the elbow and explain the rational for each test.*

- -Active range of motion
- -Resistive manual muscle testing
- -Myotome testing
- -Functional testing

- -Passive range of motion
- -Dermatome testing
- -Reflex testing

V. Multiple Choice Questions ———————————————————

Instructions: *Choose the best answer for each question.*

____1. Subjective information is gained through the _____ of the HOPS process.
   a. history
   b. observation
   c. palpation
   d. special tests

____2. The most appropriate place to perform injury assessment is:
   a. on the field
   b. in the gymnasium
   c. in the athletic training room
   d. in the classroom

____3. The heart is _____ to the abdomen.
   a. posterior
   b. superior
   c. inferior
   d. dorsal

____4. The elbow is _____ to the shoulder.
   a. proximal
   b. distal
   c. anterior
   d. superior

____5. The little finger is _____ to the thumb.
   a. medial
   b. lateral
   c. superficial
   d. proximal

____6. The direct cause of an injury is referred to as:
   a. sequela
   b. a syndrome
   c. mechanism of injury
   d. prognosis

____7. When the palm is moved in a downward position, this movement is termed:
   a. rotation
   b. flexion
   c. supination
   d. pronation

____8. Long lasting deep pain may be indicative of:
   a. a skin rash
   b. an open wound
   c. injury to bone
   d. a blister

____9. Pain that subsides during activity may be indicative of:
   a. acute injury
   b. injury to bone
   c. chronic condition or inflammation
   d. nerve injury

___10. The scan examination aids in determining:
   a. gross motor function
   b. sensation
   c. congenital abnormalities
   d. normal gait pattern

___11. Effusion is often associated with:
   a. bone injury
   b. interarticular injury
   c. extra-articular injury
   d. bruising of soft tissue

_12. To determine varus or valgus angulation of the heels, you would have to observe an athlete's posture from a/an _____ view.
a. anterior   c. posterior
b. side   d. lateral

_13. Decreased skin temperature is indicative of:
a. inflammation   c. high blood pressure
b. reduction in circulation d. muscle spasms

_14. When using a goniometer to measure joint range of motion, the stationary arm of the goniometer is placed _____ to the proximal bone of the joint being measured.
a. distal   c. lateral
b. superior   d. parallel

_15. Passive movement will determine injury to _____.
a. contractile tissue   c. muscular tissue
b. noncontractile tissue   d. ocular injuries

_16. To determine the presence of accessory movement, the joint would be manipulated in a/an _____.
a. loose packed position   c. resistive range of motion
b. closed packed position   d. active range of motion

_17. To determine sensation, you would test:
a. active range motion   c. myotomes
b. passive range of motion d. dermatomes

_18. A weakened muscle contraction may indicate:
a. hypesthesia   c. hypertrophy
b. paresis   d. paresthesia

_19. A _____ may indicate damage to a nerve root.
a. diminished tendon reflex   c. change in pulse
b. decrease in temperature   d. decrease in range of motion

_20. During an on-the-field assessment, _____ should always be ruled out before moving the injured athlete.
a. fracture   c. fracture and major ligament injury
b. major ligament injury d. bruises and skin lacerations

VI. Additional Activities

1. **Visit with a physician or physical therapist to better understand SOAP note documentation.**

2. **After performing HOPS procedure on an injured athlete, reassess the athlete using the SOAP note method.**

3. **Perform active, passive, and resistive range of motion for the elbow with a partner.**

4. **Using the shoulder and knee joint, determine loose and closed packed positions of each joint.**

Student's Key

I. Key Terms

Etiology — — — — — — The science and study of the causes of disease

Pathology — — — — — — The cause of an injury, its development, and functional changes due to the injury process

Observation — — — — — Visual analysis of overall appearance, symmetry, general motor function, posture, and gait

Inspection — — — — — — Refers to factors seen at the actual injury site, such as redness, swelling, bruising, cuts, or scars

Syndrome — — — — — — An accumulation of signs and symptoms associated with a particular injury or disease

Atrophy — — — — — — — A wasting away or deterioration of tissue

Hypertrophy — — — — — Increase in general bulk or size of an individual tissue, such as a muscle

Ecchymosis — — — — — Bruise; discoloration of the skin due to subcutaneous bleeding

Effusion — — — — — — — The escape of fluid from the blood vessels into the surrounding tissues or joint cavity

Dermatome — — — — — — Area of skin supplied by the cutaneous branches of each spinal nerve

Myotome — — — — — — A group of muscles primarily innervated by a single nerve root

Nerve root — — — — — — The portion of a nerve associated with its origin in the spinal cord, such as C_5 or L_5

Proprioceptors — — — — Specialized deep sensory nerve cells in joints, ligaments, muscles, and tendons sensitive to stretch, tension, and pressure that is responsible for position and movement

Muscle spindle — — — Encapsulated receptor found in muscle tissue sensitive to stretch

I. Key Terms (Con't)

Anesthesia — — — — — Loss of sensation

Hypesthesia — — — — — Excessive tactile sensation

Paresthesia — — — — — Abnormal sensation, such as numbness, tingling, or burning

Paresis — — — — — — Partial paralysis of a muscle leading to a weakened contraction

Referred pain — — — — Pain felt in a region of the body other than where the source or actual cause of the pain is located

Somatic pain — — — — Pain originating in the skin, ligaments, muscles, bones, or joints

Visceral pain — — — — Pain resulting from injury or disease to an organ in the thoracic or abdominal cavity

Goniometer — — — — — Protractor used to measure joint position and available joint motion (ROM)

End feel — — — — — — The sensation felt in the joint as it reaches the end of the available range of motion

Anatomical position — — Standardized position with the body erect, facing forward, with the arms at the sides and palms facing forward

Active movement — — — Joint motion performed voluntarily by the individual through muscular contractions

Passive movement — — — A limb or body part is moved through the range of motion with no assistance from the individual

Accessory movement — — Movements within a joint that cannot be voluntarily performed by the individual

Static position — — — — Stationary position in which no motion occurs

Closed packed position — Most stable joint position in which the two joint surfaces fit precisely together and supporting ligaments and capsule are maximally taut

Loose packed position — — Resting position where the joint is under the least amount of strain

I. Key Terms (Con't)

Appendicular segment — — Relates to the extremities of the body including the arms and legs

Axial segment — — — — — Central part of the body including the head and trunk

Antalgic gait — — — — — Walking with a limp

Indication — — — — — — A condition that could benefit from a specific action

Contraindication — — — — A condition adversely affected by a specific action

Modalities — — — — — — Therapeutic physical agents that promote optimal healing, such as thermotherapy, cryotherapy, electrotherapy, or manual therapy

Diagnosis — — — — — — Definitive determination of the nature of the injury or illness made only by physicians

Prognosis — — — — — — Probable course or progress of an injury or disease

Sequela — — — — — — — A condition that may follow as a consequence of an injury or disease

Painful arc — — — — — — Pain located within a limited number of degrees in the range of motion

Valgus — — — — — — — — Denoting a deformity in which the distal body part angulates away from the middle of the body

Varus — — — — — — — — Denoting a deformity in which the distal body part angulates toward the midline of the body

II. Simulations

1   Elbow Injury Assessment

(Refer to Field Strategies 4-1 on text page 110 and 4-2 on text page 115)

Did you ask subjective information to determine a history of the elbow injury?
- primary complaint; current nature, location, and onset of condition
- mechanism of injury; how did the condition occur and when did it occur
- extent of pain or disability due to injury; sport and nonsport participation activities
- type of pain; stabbing, aching, radiating, intermittent, how long does the pain last, what aggravates or alleviates pain
- type of symptoms; location, onset, severity, frequency and duration
- previous injuries to the area
- related medical history
- previous treatment and use of medications

1A. Did you observe and bilaterally inspect for the following?
- consciousness and body language
- individual's willingness to move
- scan examination
- deformity
- swelling
- discoloration
- scars that might indicate previous surgery

1B. Did you palpate bilaterally for:
- temperature
- swelling
- point tenderness
- crepitus
- deformity
- muscle spasm
- cutaneous sensation
- pulse

1C. Did you perform the following special tests bilaterally?
- active and passive elbow movement
- resisted manual muscle testing of the elbow musculature
- neurological testing
- stress testing for elbow ligamentous integrity
- functional testing

1   Elbow Injury Assessment (Con't)

1D. If you recognized the tennis player's injury as a mild muscle strain of the wrist extensors, you are correct. Pain and weakness have affected normal activities of daily living, but no joint instability is present. This individual does not need to see a physician at this time but needs an appropriate treatment and rehabilitation program.

1E. Did you have the tennis player perform the sport skills associated with tennis (forehand, serve, backhand) at low intensity and frequency progressing to higher intensity and frequency?

2   Low Back Pathology Assessment

(Refer to Field Strategy 4-3 on page 117 in the text)

Did your scan examination include gross motor movements of the neck, trunk, and extremities such as:
   - looking up at the ceiling, looking down, and neck rotation
   - forward bending and trunk rotation
   - straight leg raises

2A. Did your postural examination include observation of:
   - spinal curve abnormalities
   - anterior, posterior, and lateral views of the body looking for proper alignment of anatomical structures
   - general symmetry of the shoulders, hips, and knees

III. Situations

l. Directional Terms - (Refer to Table 4-1 on pages 106 to 107 in the text) - When you reported the location of the pain to the school nurse, did you use directional and anatomical terms such as 2 inches proximal to the elbow joint particularly on the medial aspect of the humerus?

2. Anatomical Position - Did you instruct the individual to stand erect facing forward with the arms at the side of the body with the palms facing forward?

3. Pain Assessment - (Refer to Table 4-2 on page 114 in the text) - Did you determine the type and degree of pain by asking the golfer the following questions:

III. Situations (Con't)

Is the pain:
- constant or intermittent
- dull or sharp
- radiating or referred
- localized or diffused
- bothersome after activity, during activity, or all the time
- does it wake them up at night

Does rest help relieve the pain? What activities increase/decrease the pain? How long does the pain last?

Using a scale of 1 to 10 with 10 being severe, when the pain begins, how severe is it and how long does it usually last?

4. Related Medical History - To obtain a related medical history on the runner, did you ask if the runner had any previous:
- respiratory or vascular problems
- heat illness
- seizures
- chronic medical problems
- loss of consciousness or head injuries

5. Vascular and Nerve Assessment - (Refer to Figure 4-18 on page 127 in the text) - To rule out major artery involvement with the football player's shoulder injury, did you check for a distal radial pulse?

To rule out nerve involvement, did you test cutaneous sensation by assessing dermatome function. Did you:
- ask the individual to close both eyes.
- run your fingers along both sides of the arm and shoulder and ask if it feels the same on both sides
- complete this same procedure on the uninjured shoulder and arm

6. Elbow Range of Motion - (Refer to Figure 4-15 on page 122 in the text) - To determine elbow range of motion subjectively, did you have the athlete perform elbow flexion and extension and compare the motions bilaterally?

To determine elbow range of motion objectively, did you use a goniometer? Did they:
- place the stationary arm parallel to the proximal bone
- coincide the axis of the goniometer with the joint axis of the elbow
- place the moving arm parallel to the distal bone

III. Situations (Con't)

7. Myotome Testing - (Refer to Tables 4-6 on page 126 in the text and 4-7 on page 128 in the text) - Because there was no pain on resisted manual muscle testing but there was weakness, did you determine that this could indicate nerve involvement and that the individual should be referred to a physician for further evaluation?

8. Reflex Testing - (Refer to Table 4-8 on page 129 in the text) - To determine central nervous system damage by way of reflex testing for the low back injury, did you test the deep tendon patella reflex knee jerk? To perform the knee jerk reflex test, you should strike the patella tendon with a reflex hammer. Deep tendon reflexes tend to be diminished or absent when the specific nerve root being tested is damaged.

9. SOAP Notes - (Refer to Table 4-9 on page 132 in the text) - Did you determine that it is extremely important for all employees to use a uniform method of documentation to verify services rendered and to record patient evaluation, progress, and assessment, particularly when numerous individuals are involved in the patient's rehabilitation program? Did you provide the SOAP note format for a record-keeping method?

IV. Special Tests

Refer to pages 119–130 in the text.

V. Multiple Choice Answers

1. a	8. c	15. b
2. c	9. c	16. a
3. b	10. a	17. d
4. b	11. b	18. b
5. a	12. c	19. a
6. c	13. b	20. ?
7. d	14. d	

Chapter 5: Therapeutic Exercise and Therapeutic Modalities

After completing this chapter you should be able to:

- Identify the five theoretical emotional stages an individual progresses through when confronted with a disabling injury

- Identify and describe the process in designing a therapeutic exercise program

- Explain the four phases of therapeutic exercise programs, goals, and methodology of implementation

- List the criteria used to clear an individual to return to full participation in sport

- Describe the major groups of modalities, indications and contraindications for their use, and their application to manage inflammation and promote healing

- Describe how nutrition can enhance healing

I. Key Terms

Instructions: *On a separate sheet of paper define the following terms.*

Indication	Iontophoresis	Hypomobility
Contraindication	Therapeutic drugs	Hypermobility
Cryotherapy	Analgesic	Overload principle
Cryokinetics	Analgesic effect	Agonist
Cold allergies	Anesthetics	Antagonist
Hunting response	Antipyresis	Strength
Thermotherapy	Counterirritant	Muscular power
Hyperemia	Salicylates	Muscular endurance
Wheal	Contracture	Sticking point
Current	Flexibility	Kinetics
Voltage	Ballistic stretching	Kinematic chains
Cathode	Static stretching	Plyometric training
Anode	Active inhibition	Coordination
Cavitation	Reciprocal inhibition	Raynaud's phenomenon
Phonophoresis	Proprioceptive neuromuscular facilitation	Valsalva effect

II. Simulations

Instructions: *Perform the following simulated experiences.*

 A basketball player has sustained a season-ending knee injury. How might this individual psychologically react to this injury? What impact might the player's feelings have on his/her motivation to recover from this injury?

1A. The basketball player is depressed and refuses to accept that the injury is season ending. What can you do to help the basketball player overcome these feelings and other emotions that might hinder his/her progress in the therapeutic exercise and rehabilitation program?

 A lacrosse player has sustained an acromioclavicular sprain of the shoulder and is now ready to begin therapeutic exercise. What is the first step the athletic trainer must perform to initiate the rehabilitation process? How does the trainer accomplish this using the SOAP note format?

2A. Now that you have recorded the objective portion of the SOAP note, develop a therapeutic exercise program for the lacrosse player by performing the A portion of the SOAP note format.

2B. You have now assessed the patient and have developed both long- and short-term goals. It is now time to develop the treatment plan or the P portion of the SOAP notes. Demonstrate how you will do this.

 A gymnast has sustained a sprained ankle. Demonstrate Phase I of the therapeutic exercise program.

3A. The acute inflammatory symptoms have been controlled using the PRICE principles. Demonstrate what exercises can be used to increase range of motion of the injured ankle and enhance healing.

3B. You and the gymnast are having a difficult time in achieving increased ankle range of motion. What might be causing this inhibition?

3 (Con't)
A gymnast has sustained a sprained ankle. Demonstrate Phase I of the therapeutic exercise program.

3C. The gymnast has regained pain-free range of motion of the injured ankle joint. Can the gymnast return to practice at this time? Why? Does the gymnast need to continue the rehabilitation process? If yes, explain and demonstrate what the gymnast will be doing in the next phase of the rehabilitation program.

3D. The gymnast has completed Phase III of the rehabilitation process and is ready to return to activity. Explain and demonstrate how the gymnast will functionally return to activity.

3E. What criteria will be used to determine if the gymnast is ready to return to full activity and competition?

3F. During the rehabilitation process, should the gymnast be concerned about nutrition and diet? Why?

A runner has sustained a stress fracture of the foot. The physician suggests no weight-bearing activity for 1 week. Explain and demonstrate how to fit the runner with crutches.

4A. After two days of being on crutches, the runner is getting aggravated and bored. What type of activity can the athlete do to maintain cardiovascular conditioning and relieve boredom?

III. Situations

Instructions: *Work with a partner to cooperatively analyze and answer the following situations.*

1. A tennis player has sustained a mild chronic strain to the wrist extensors. What long- and short-term goals might you and the player establish for the therapeutic exercise program?

2. A wrestler has been in a therapeutic exercise program for the past month for a shoulder injury. How is progress monitored in the program? What techniques may be used to motivate the individual to work harder?

III. Situations (Con't)

3. A diver hit a foot on the board and you have applied the PRICE principle. What are the concepts behind the PRICE principle, and why is it used with an acute injury?

4. A hurdler sustained a strain to a hamstring muscle. There are no available modalities to use to decrease the muscle spasm and to assist in muscle relaxation. Without the availability of therapeutic modalities, explain and demonstrate how the athlete can relax the hamstring muscle.

5. After working on range of motion for several days, a baseball pitcher is having problems regaining active elbow flexion. Full flexion, however, can be gained through passive means. What can the pitcher do to achieve active full flexion?

6. A group of dancers has been doing ballistic stretching for years. What strategies can you use to explain that ballistic stretching is actually detrimental to flexibility and that static stretching is more optimal? Explain the guidelines used while doing static stretching.

7. The punter on the football team wants to increase flexibility of the hamstrings. Explain and demonstrate how proprioceptive neuromuscular facilitation (PNF) stretching can help accomplish this.

8. You are a high school athletic trainer with a limited budget. What type of rehabilitative equipment can you purchase to increase muscle strength, endurance, and power without overextending your budget?

9. A basketball player has sustained a quadriceps strain and is now in Phase III of the rehabilitation process. Explain and demonstrate what exercises can be used to increase muscular power?

10. A running back has undergone surgery to repair a menisci injury. The supervising physician has suggested closed chain exercises. Why? Explain and demonstrate a few closed chain exercises that could be used in a lower extremity program.

ll. A recreational sport participant has sustained a strained calf muscle. You want to increase the range of motion of the calf muscle. What type of cryotherapy technique could be used prior to stretching to facilitate the stretching program? Why are these effective?

12. A volleyball player sustained a jammed finger and is in Phase II of the therapeutic exercise program. What type of thermotherapy program can be used to supplement the program? How will you administer this modality?

III. Situations (Con't)

13. A baseball player is suffering from chronic biceps tendinitis. The physician has recommended a modality that will produce a deep thermal effect. What modality will you choose? Why? What contraindications must you be aware of prior to applying this type of treatment? Are there any medications that a physician might prescribe for this injury?

14. A shot putter has strained a triceps muscle. After applying the PRICE principle, what other modality can be combined with PRICE to decrease pain, muscle spasms, and edema? Are there any over-the-counter medications that might aid in this process?

15. A swimmer is recovering from shoulder surgery. You want to use massage to help break up soft tissue adhesions left from the surgical procedure. What massage technique will assist in achieving this goal? Why?

16. A golfer is experiencing acute low back muscle spasms. What type of treatment or medication will be best for the golfer to relieve the muscle spasms?

17. A wrestler wants a good nutritional program to use while training and competing. What guidelines can be provided to this athlete to ensure safe weight loss or weight gain?

IV. Multiple Choice Questions

Instructions: *Choose the best answer for each question.*

___1. Biofeedback techniques and transcendental meditation are used to:
    a. decrease painful muscle spasms   c. supplement strength training
    b. promote generalized body relaxation   d. enhance motivation

___2. Documentation of mechanism of injury, signs and symptoms, and level of dysfunction is part of the _____ portion of the SOAP note documentation.
    a. objective   c. subjective
    b. assessment   d. planning

___3. Developing a problem list of the athlete's injury is part of the _____ portion of the SOAP note documentation.
    a. objective   c. assessment
    b. subjective   d. planning

___4. Long-term goals specifically focus on:
    a. daily exercise protocol
    b. deficits in sport-specific skills
    c. deficits in activities of daily living and sport-specific skills
    d. specific components of skill development

____5. The major goal in Phase I of the rehabilitation process is to:
   a. evaluate the injury
   b. control the inflammatory reponse
   c. regain deficits in range of motion
   d. regain deficits in functional activity

____6. Immobilization of a joint for _____may lead to joint adhesions that inhibit muscle fiber regeneration.
   a. 5 days
   b. less than 2 weeks
   c. 10 to 14 days
   d. more than 2 weeks

____7. Application of cold immediately following an injury leads to:
   a. vasodilation
   b. vasoconstriction
   c. increased nerve impulses
   d. increased time for blood coagulation

____8. Continuous passive motion is used to:
   a. prevent joint adhesions
   b. decrease swelling
   c. decrease muscle spasms
   d. enhance strength

____9. _____law states that when a muscle is contracting, its corresponding antagonistic muscle is inhibited, and thus relaxed. This law is a basis of Jacobson's system of progressive relaxation.
   a. Wolff's
   b. Cosine
   c. Sherrington's
   d. SAID

___10. An athlete can move into Phase III of the rehabilitation process when all but the following criteria have been completed.
   a. passive and active range of motion are within 80% of normal in the unaffected limb
   b. inflammation is persistent
   c. joint flexibility in the affected limb is restored as compared to unaffected limb
   d. cardiovascular endurance and general body strength are maintained at preinjury level

___11. The _____causes a reflex inhibition in the antagonist muscle and protects the musculotendinous unit from excessive tensile forces.
   a. Golgi tendon organ
   b. muscle spindles
   c. tendon sheath
   d. proprioceptors

___12. Strength gains depend primarily on:
   a. the specific training method
   b. duration of the exercise session
   c. intensity of the overload
   d. frequence of the exercise session

___13. Contractions performed every 20 degrees throughout the available range of motion are called:
   a. multiple-angle isotonic exercises
   b. mutiple-angle isometric exercises
   c. isometric exercises
   d. isokinetic exercises

___14. An athlete is performing a bicep curl as an exercise for a bicep strain. This exercise is considered to be:
   a. an isometric exercise
   b. open chain exercise
   c. closed chain exercise
   d. isokinetic exercise

__15. Closed chain exercises are recommended for several reasons. One of these reasons is:
a. closed chain exercises increase strength at a faster rate than open chain
b. closed chain exercises increase range of motion faster
c. closed chain exercises reduce shearing forces about the joint
d. closed chain exercises facilitate the inflammatory response

__16. A biomechanical ankle platform system is often used to:
a. increase range of motion
b. decrease swelling
c. improve sensory cues and balance of upper extremity
d. improve sensory cues and balance of lower extremity

__17. The _____hypothesizes that cold inhibits pain transmission by stimulating large diameter neurons in the spinal cord.
a. Sherrington's law
b. Wolff's law
c. Gate theory of pain
d. Hunting response

__18. Because of hyperemia occurring after an ice massage treatment has ended, it is not recommended for:
a. acute injuries
b. chronic injuries
c. muscular injuries
d. older patients

__19. A modality that is often used to increase range of motion prior to exercise is:
a. cold whirlpools
b. ice massage
c. hydrocollator packs
d. vapocoolant sprays

__20. To reduce swelling, all of the following modalities could be used except:
a. neuromuscular electrical stimulation
b. contrast baths
c. paraffin bath
d. cryotherapy

__21. _____ is a medium that conducts or facilitates the movement of ions.
a. skin
b. water
c. fat
d. lotion

__22. A galvanic current is a/an _____ type of electrical current.
a. alternating
b. faradic
c. direct
d. pulsed

__23. The _____occurs when a current reaches the threshold whereby ions are transferred through nerve and muscle fibers to cause an electrical impulse or muscle contraction.
a. overload principle
b.gate-control pain theory
c. all-or-none response
d. electrical stimulation principle

__24. Direct current is primarily used to do all of the following but:
a. reeducate muscles
b. stimulate denervated muscle
c. enhance wound healing
d. during iontophoresis

__25. Transcutaneous electrical nerve stimulation is used to:
a. decrease acute and chonic pain
b. decrease chronic pain
c. decrease muscle spasms
d. reeducate muscular tissue

__26. All of the following are nonsteroidal anti-inflammatory drugs but:
a. acetylsalicylic acid
b. Indocin
c. Advil
d. Flexeril

___27. Local anesthetics eliminate _____ by blocking afferent neural transmissions along peripheral nerves.

a. long-term pain   c. sensory function

b. short-term pain   d. muscle spasms

___28. Acetaminophin reduces pain and fever but has no appreciable _____.

a. analgesic effects

b. anticoagulant effects

c. anti-inflammatory effects

d. anti-inflammatory and anticoagulant effects

___29. Skeletal muscle relaxants are used to:

a. produce analgesia   c. relieve muscle spasms

b. produce anesthesia   d. increase muscle excitability

___30. Diets should be high in _____ and low in _____.

a. protein and low in fats and carbohydrates

b. fruits, vegetables, and breads and low in fats and sugar

c. breads and pasta and low in fruits and vegetables

d. carbohydrates and low in protein and sugar

V. Additional Activities

1. With a partner, practice applying various modalities to each other.

2. Visit a physical therapy center and observe the various types of modalities and rehabilitation equipment used in patient care.

3. Visit a pharmacist to inquire about the various over-the-counter and prescription drugs used for athletic injuries.

4. Design a rehabilitation program for an athlete who has sustained a moderate ankle sprain.

5. Visit with a certified athletic trainer who has an isokinetic device (kin-kom, cybex, biodex) and inquire about its use during rehabilitation and testing of athletic injuries.

6. Visit a strength and conditioning coach and inquire about his or her role in the rehabilitation process.

7. Design a functional progression program for a basketball player who has sustained a knee injury.

I. Key Terms

Indication — — — — — —   A condition that could benefit from use of a specific modality

Contraindication — — —   A condition adversely affected if a particular modality is used

Cryotherapy — — — — —   Cold application

Cryokinetics — — — — —   Use of cold treatments prior to an exercise session

Cold allergies — — — — —   Hypersensitivity to cold, leading to superficial vascular reaction manifested by transient itching, erythema, hives, or whitish swellings (wheals)

Wheals — — — — — — —   A smooth, slightly elevated area on the body that appears red or white and is accompanied by severe itching; commonly seen in allergies to mechanical or chemical irritants

Hunting response — — —   Cyclical periods of vasoconstriction and vasodilation after ice application

Thermotherapy — — — —   Heat applications

Hyperemia — — — — — —   Increase of blood flow into a region once treatment has ended

Current — — — — — — —   The actual movement of ions

Voltage — — — — — — —   The force that causes the ions to move

Cathode — — — — — — —   Negatively charged electrode in a direct current system

Anode — — — — — — —   Positively charged electrode in a direct current system

Cavitation — — — — — —   Gas bubble formation due to nonthermal effects of ultrasound

Phonophoresis — — — —   The introduction of anti-inflammatory drugs through the skin with the use of ultrasound

I. Key Terms (Con't)

Iontophoresis — — — — — Technique whereby direct current is used to drive charged molecules from certain medications into damaged tissue

Therapeutic drugs — — — Prescription or over-the-counter medications used to treat an injury or illness

Analgesic — — — — — A drug or agent that reduces the response to pain and is usually accompanied by sedation without loss of consciousness

Analgesic effect — — — — Condition whereby pain is not perceived, such as in a numbing or sedative effect

Anesthetics — — — — — A drug or agent that leads to an inability to perceive pain and/or other sensations

Antipyresis — — — — — — Action whereby body temperature associated with a fever is reduced

Counterirritant — — — — A substance causing irritation of superficial sensory nerves that reduces pain transmission from another underlying irritation

Salicylates — — — — — Any salt or salicylic acid; used in aspirin

Contracture — — — — — Adhesions occurring in an immobilized muscle leading to an shortened contractile state

Flexibility — — — — — Total range of motion at a joint dependent on normal joint mechanics, mobility of soft tissue, and muscle extensibility

Ballistic stretching — — — Increasing flexibility by utilizing repetitive bouncing motions at the end of the available range of motion

Static stretching — — — — Slow and deliberate muscle stretching used to increase flexibility

Active inhibition — — — Technique whereby an individual consciously relaxes a muscle prior to stretching

Reciprocal inhibition — — Technique using an active contraction of the agonist to cause a reflex relaxation in the antagonist, allowing it to stretch; a phenomenon resulting from reciprocal innervation

I. Key Terms (Con't)

Proprioceptive — — — — — Exercises that stimulate proprioceptors in muscles, tendons,
neuromuscular facilitation   and joints to improve flexibility and strength

Hypomobility — — — — — Decreased motion at a joint

Hypermobility — — — — — Increased motion at a joint; joint laxity

Overload principle — — — Physiologic improvements occur only when an individual
physically demands more of the muscle than is normally
required

Agonist — — — — — — — A muscle that performs the desired movement; a primary mover

Antagonist — — — — — — A muscle that acts in opposition to another muscle; its agonist

Strength — — — — — — — The ability of a muscle to produce resulting force in one
maximal effort, either statically or dynamically

Muscular power — — — — The ability of muscles to produce force in a given unit of
time

Muscular endurance — — — The ability of muscles to exert tension over an extended
period of time

Sticking point — — — — — Presence of insufficient strength to move a body segment
through a particular angle

Kinetics — — — — — — — The study of forces that affect motion

Kinematic chains — — — — A series of interrelated joints that constitute a complex motor
unit so that motion at one joint will produce motion at the
other joints in a predictable manner

Plyometric training — — — Exercises that employ explosive movements to develop
muscular power

Coordination — — — — — The body's ability to execute smooth, accurate, and
controlled movements

Raynaud's phenomenon — Intermittent bilateral attacks of ischemia in the digits,
marked by severe pallor, burning, and pain brought on by cold

Valsalva effect — — — — — Holding one's breath against a closed glottis, resulting in
sharp increases in blood pressure

II. Simulations

 Psychological Needs

Did you use Kubler-Ross's six theoretical emotional stages an individual progresses through when confronted with grief to describe how the individual might react psychologically toward the knee injury?
- denial of the injury
- isolation of self from the team
- anger with self
- bargaining
- depression
- acceptance of injury

Did you determine that the emotions experienced by the individual might decrease the motivation to progress through treatment, rehabilitation and full return to activity?

lA. To help the basketball player deal with depression and other emotions experienced during the injury, did your plan include:
- reasoning with the individual to convince him/her that the injury is real and that further participation could lead to further injury and/or disability
- if the individual becomes angry, allow him/her to have space to vent frustrations
- motivate the individual to continue being part of the team by arranging many of the treatment and rehabilitation in the same area that the team is practicing
- develop realistic short-term goals with the player
- demonstrate progress through the use of charts and graphs on a continual basis

 Designing an Individualized Therapeutic Exercise Program

(Refer to Table 5-2 on page 141 in the text)

Did you determine that the first step in designing a therapeutic exercise program for the injured tennis player was to do a patient assessment? Following the SOAP note format did your assessment include documentation of:
- mechanism of injury
- signs and symptoms
- dysfunction as compared to the noninjured body part

2A. The A portion of the SOAP note format is assessment. Did your assessment include:
- analyzing and interpreting information gained in the subjective and objective portions of the SOAP notes
- identification of specific deficits and assets
- recording specific problems in a section called the problem list

2B. Did your treatment plan include the four phases of rehabilitation that comprise the therapeutic exercise program?
- Phase I controlling the inflammatory response, pain, swelling, and ecchymosis and patient education
- Phase II regains any deficits in active and passive range of motion at the affected joint
- Phase III regains muscle strength, endurance, and power in the affected limb
- Phase IV prepares the individual to return to activity and includes analysis of motion, sport specific skill training, regaining coordination, and improving cardiovascular conditioning

3 Ankle Sprain

(Refer to Field Strategies 5-l on page 143 in the text; 5-4 on page 148 in the text; and 5-ll on page 164 in the text)

In Phase I did you:
- control swelling at the ankle by applying PRICE
- choose either intermittent compression, electrical muscle stimulation, or TENS as modalities to help control hemorrhage, eliminate edema, and control pain
- protect and restrict activity at the ankle by immobilization through the use of an elastic wrap, tape, brace, and/or crutches

3A. To achieve an increase in range of motion did you:
- remove the ankle brace or splint prior to beginning exercises
- have the athlete perform both active and passive range of motion exercises as tolerated in plantar flexion, dorsiflexion, inversion, and eversion
- depending on the inflammatory response, use thermotherapy (warm whirlpool), cryotherapy, and/or electrical muscle stimulation prior to range of motion exercises
- use a cryokenetic program
- apply ice after exercise session

3B. Did you determine that the following factors could inhibit joint range of motion?
- bony block
- joint adhesions
- muscle tightness
- tight skin or inelastic scar tissue
- swelling or pain

3C. No, the gymnast cannot return to activity because of the risk of possible reinjury to the ankle. The gymnast must restrengthen the muscles surrounding the ankle joint and move into Phase III of the rehabilitation process. The gymnast may, however, practice certain skills at low intensity if the ankle is not placed at risk for reinjury.

Did Phase III include:
- the overload principle to increase muscular strength, endurance, and power
- use of the specific adaptations to imposed demands (SAID) principle
- isometric, isotonic, and isokinetic exercises
- closed chain exercises

3D. Did Phase IV (return to activity) of the gymnast's ankle rehabilitation program include:
- muscle strength assessment
- correction of biomechanical inefficiencies
- restoration of coordination, muscle strength, endurance, and power in sport specific skills
- improved cardiovascular endurance
- progressively increase in intensity and duration of activities

3E. Did your criteria for the gymnast to return to activity and competition include:
- normal biomechanical function of sport specific functional patterns
- muscle strength, endurance, and power in affected limb equal to that of the unaffected limb
- normal balance and coordination
- cardiovascular endurance at or greater than preinjury level
- wearing of appropriate taping or bracing if needed
- medical clearance from supervising physician

3 Ankle Sprain (Con't)

3F. Yes, the gymnast should be concerned about his/her diet during the rehabilitation process. An injured individual must have an adequate diet that provides the nutrients necessary to enhance wound healing (carbohydrates, fats, proteins, water, vitamins, and minerals). In addition, a diet high in carbohydrates should supply the energy necessary to train and compete on a highly competitive level.

4 Stress Fracture

(Refer to Field Strategies 5-2 on page 144 in the text and 5-9 on page 160 in the text)

Did you use the following guidelines to fit crutches for the runner?
- have the individual stand erect in low-heeled shoes
- place the tip of the crutch slightly in front of and to the side of the involved leg
- adjust the length so that the axillary pad is l to l 1/2 inches below the axilla
- adjust the hand grips so the elbow is flexed at about 30 degrees and is at the level of the greater trochanter.

4A. Did you suggest that the runner choose one of the following cardiovascular programs to do while in the nonweight-bearing phase of their injury?
- upper body ergometer
- cycling
- rowing
- swimming

III. Situations

l. Long- and Short-Term Goals - (Refer to pages 139–140 in the text and Table 5-l on text page 140) - Did the long-term goals for the tennis player include:
- pain-free bilateral range of motion
- bilateral muscular strength, endurance, and power
- maintenance of cardiovascular endurance
- restoration of normal joint biomechanics
- increased proprioception and kinesthetic awareness
- restoration of bilateral function of activities of daily living (ADL)
- pain-free unlimited motion in tennis skills with the use of a tennis elbow support

III. Situations (Con't)

1. Long- and Short-Term Goals (Con't) - Did the short-term goals include:
- control inflammation, pain, and swelling
- restore active range and passive range of motion as tolerated
- protect the area and decrease level of activity
- maintain wrist and shoulder strength
- maintain cardiovascular endurance with weight-bearing exercise

2. Monitoring Progress - To monitor the progress of the wrestler did you include the following parameters?
- daily documentation of exercise program
- documentation of edema, hemorrhaging, muscle spasms, atrophy, and infection that might impede the healing process
- periodical measurements of girth, range of motion, muscular strength, endurance, power, and cardiovascular fitness
- reevaluation of exercise program based on documentation

3. PRICE - (Refer to Field Strategy 5-l on page 143 in the text) - Did your rationale for applying the PRICE principle to the acutely injured diver's foot include:
- protecting and restricting activity decreases the chance of further injury and is essential if repair and healing are to progress in a timely manner
- ice leads to vasoconstriction, decreased circulation and capillary permeability, and decreased time for blood coagulation
- compression assists in decreasing hemorrhage and hematoma formation
- elevation uses gravity to reduce pooling of fluids and pressure inside the venous and lymphatic vessels to prevent fluid from filtering into the surrounding tissue spaces

4. Specific Muscle Relaxation - (Refer to Field Strategy 5-3 on page 145 in the text) - Did you use Jacobson's relaxation exercises to help the hurdler relax the hamstring muscles? Did you:
- focus on the hamstring while initiating an isometric contraction of the hamstring for five to seven seconds
- relax the hamstring while imagining the muscle is heavy, warm, and relaxed after the contraction
- if continued muscle tension is perceived, repeat the process

5. Active Assistive Range of Motion - Did you determine that the baseball pitcher must use active assistive range of motion exercises to achieve full elbow flexion? Did you assist in moving the elbow through the available pain-free motion?

III. Situations (Con't)

6. Ballistic and Static Stretching - (Refer to text pages 149–150 and Field Strategy 5-5 on page 150 in the text) - Did your rationale include:
- ballistic stretching uses repetitive bouncing motions at the end of the available range of motion that causes muscle spindles to repetitively stretch, but since the bouncing motions are so short in duration, the Golgi tendon organs do not fire. As such, the muscles resist relaxation.
- ballistic stretching often enhances muscles to remain contracted to prevent overstretching, leading to microscopic tears in the musculotendinous unit
- in a static stretch, movement is slow and deliberate. The Golgi tendon organs are able to override impulses from the muscle spindles, leading to a safer and more effective muscle stretch

Static stretching guidelines suggest that:
- muscle is stretched to a point where a mild burn is felt
- this position is maintained statically for about 15 seconds and repeated several times

7. PNF Stretching - (Refer to Field Strategy 5-6 on page 151 in the text) - Did you choose to use the contract-relax technique of PNF stretching that includes:
- passively stretching the hamstring muscle and then asking the individual to contract the hamstring against an isometric resistance applied by you for 3, 6, or 10 seconds followed by a relaxation period.
- alternating contractions and passive stretching repeating the process five to eight times

8. Resistance Equipment - Did you determine that free weights, theraband, elastic, and surgical tubing can be purchased relatively inexpensively to assist in Phase III of the rehabilitation process?

9. Plyometric Training - (Refer to Field Strategy 5-7 on page 156 in the text) - Did you choose plyometric training to increase the volleyball player's muscular endurance? Did your plyometric program include:
- progressive intensity and frequency in exercises
- exercises such as standing jumps, multiple jumps, depth jumps, bounding, and leaping
- performing exercises on grass or other resilient surfaces
- performing exercises every 3 days to allow for recovery

10. Closed Chain Exercises - Reasons why closed chain exercises are recommended include:
- multiple joints can be exercised through weight-bearing and muscular co-contractions
- velocity and torque are more controlled
- shear forces are reduced
- proprioceptors are reeducated
- postural and stabilization mechanics are facilitated
- exercises can work in spiral or diagonal movement patterns

Did you include the following closed chain exercises as example exercises for the running back?
- flat foot exercises
- Profitter exercises
- BAPS or wobble board exercises
- sand walking exercises
- balancing on toes exercises

11. Ice Massage - Did you choose to use ice massage on the strained calf muscle? Ice massage is useful for its analgesic effect in relieving pain that may inhibit stretching of a muscle and has been shown to decrease muscle soreness when combined with stretching.

12. Paraffin Bath - Did you choose a paraffin bath as a thermotherapy modality for the volleyball player's finger? Did the administration of the paraffin bath include:
- cleansing and removing all jewelry from the body part
- dipping the body part into the bath several times, each time allowing the previous coat to dry
- after dipping, wrap the body part in a plastic bag or towel
- elevate for 15 to 20 minutes

13. Ultrasound Application - (Refer to Table 5-6 on page 172 in the text) - Did you choose to use ultrasound for the baseball player's biceps tendinitis since ultrasound provides thermal effects and is used when a deep elevated tissue temperature is needed?

III. Situations (Con't)

Did contraindications for the use of ultrasound include:
- acute and postacute hemorrhage
- infection
- over areas of impaired circulation or sensation
- over epiphyseal growth plates or stress fracture sites
- over the pelvic area in a pregnant or menstruating female
- over the eyes, heart, spine, or genitals

Did you suggest that a physician might prescribe a prescription NSAID for the baseball player such as Indocin, Feldene, or Clinoril?

14. High-Voltage Electrical Muscle Stimulation - (Refer to Table 5-7 on page 174 in the text) - Did you choose to use high-voltage electrical muscle stimulation for the shot putter's triceps strain in conjunction with the PRICE principle? A nonsteroidal anti-inflammatory drug such as ibuprofen (Advil, Nuprin, or Motrin) may help the shot putter's condition but should not be used for a prolonged period of time.

15. Low Back Muscle Spasms - Did you use ice and high-voltage electrical muscle stimulation to treat the golfer's low back spasms? Did you suspect the physician would prescribe a skeletal muscle relaxant such as Flexeril, Soma, or Dantrium to help relieve the muscle spasms?

16. Petrissage - (Refer to Field Strategy 5-13 on page 178 in the text) - Did you choose to use petrissage on the swimmer's shoulder? Petrissage is used to break up adhesions within underlying tissues, loosen fibrous tissue, and increase elasticity of the skin.

17. Nutrition - Did you suggest the wrestler adopt the food pyramid guide for a daily diet that includes:
- 6 to 11 servings in the bread, cereal, rice, and pasta group
- 2 to 4 servings of fruit
- 3 to 5 servings of vegetables
- 2 to 3 servings in the milk, yogurt, and cheese group
- 2 to 3 servings of meat, poultry, fish, dry beans, eggs, and nuts
- limited use of fats, oils, and sweets

IV. Multiple Choice Answers

1. b	11. a	21. b
2. a	12. c	22. c
3. c	13. b	23. c
4. c	14. b	24. a
5. b	15. c	25. a
6. d	16. d	26. d
7. b	17. c	27. b
8. a	18. a	28. d
9. c	19. c	29. c
10. b	20. c	30. b

Chapter 6 Protective Equipment

After completing this chapter you should be able to:

- Identify the principles used to design protective equipment

- Explain the types of materials used in the development of padding

- List the organizations responsible for establishing standards for protective equipment

- Fit selected equipment (i.e., football helmets, mouthguards, and shoulder pads)

- Identify and discuss common protective equipment for the head and face, torso, and upper and lower body

I. Key Terms

Instructions: *On a separate sheet of paper define the following terms.*

In vivo
Prophylactic
Diffuse injury

Focal injury
Resilience

High-density material
Low-density material

II. Simulations

Instructions: *Perform the following simulated experiences.*

1 A pitcher was struck by a hard driven baseball to the right thigh. What type of injury do you suspect and what type of force caused this injury?

1A. What is your immediate treatment for this injury and what type of padding will you use to best protect the thigh from another single blow?

2 You are concerned about the various oral injuries that have occurred on your school's basketball teams. What rationale can be used to convince the coach and administration to purchase mouthguards for the teams?

2A. The administration has agreed with you to purchase mouthguards for the basketball teams. What type will you purchase? What guidelines should be used to fit the mouthguards?

III. Situations

Instructions: *Work with a partner to cooperatively analyze and answer the following situations.*

l. Preseason football camp has just begun. Explain and demonstrate what guidelines should be used to properly fit a football helmet?

2. After fitting the football helmet, what guidelines should be used to fit the shoulder pads for the football player?

3. A cyclist wants to purchase a helmet and asks for advise. What advise can you provide?

4. An individual has sustained an eye injury. The physician suggests that eye protection should be worn during sport participation. What type of eye protection should be recommended?

5. A swimmer wears soft contact lenses. What concerns would exist if the swimmer insists on wearing the contact lenses during swimming?

6. A female complains of breast pain during running. After completing a history, you find no evidence of injury. She wears a size C cup. You suspect that her pain is a result of wearing a nonsupportive bra. What suggestions will you give the runner about purchasing a sport bra?

7. A recreational softball player has sustained a moderate anterior cruciate knee sprain and has moderate instability. The attending physician suggests the athlete wear a functional knee brace when the athlete returns to activity. What type of knee brace should the individual wear and why?

8. It has been decided that all soccer players on the county's recreational teams wear shinguards. What type of material should the shinguards be made of and why?

9. A baseball player has a chronic ankle sprain that requires external support. What method of support can provide a higher level of protection for this player in all four motions? In inversion and eversion? Should the baseball player be required to follow a rehabilitation program to strengthen the muscles while using the external supportive device?

10. You are working in a sports medicine clinic as a clinical athletic trainer. During a visit to the YWCA, a woman approaches you concerning how to purchase a pair of athletic shoes. She reports having high arches and enjoys playing tennis. What guidelines will you suggest for this individual?

IV. Multiple Choice Questions

Instructions: Choose the best answer for each question.

___1. An example of a high-velocity, low-mass force in sports is:
    a. an athlete falling on an outstretched arm
    b. an athlete being struck by a baseball
    c. a running back being tackled
    d. a hockey player being checked into the sideboards

___2. All but which of the following are examples of low-density materials?
    a. orthoplast   c. foam
    b. neoprene   d. moleskin

___3. An athlete has sustained a severe bruise to the hip bone. What type of material should be used to protect this area?
    a. highly resilient material   c. low-density material
    b. nonresilient or slow recovery materials   d. neoprene insulated material

___4. The ____designs standards for football helmets.
    a. ASTM   c. HECC
    b. NCAA   d. NOCSAE

___5. When fitting a football helmet, the face mask should extend ____away from the forehead.
    a. 3/4 inches   c. two finger widths
    b. one finger width   d. 3 inches

___6. Softball and baseball helmets must:
    a. be high in resiliency   c. be easily removable for base running
    b. be a bright color   d. must be a double ear-flap design

___7. The effectiveness of a football face guard depends on all of the following but:
    a. two-point chin strap   c. helmet attachments
    b. four-point chin strap   d. strength of the face guard itself

___8. An intraoral mouthguard and tooth protector is required in all interscholastic and intercollegiate sports but which of the following:
    a. basketball   c. football
    b. field hockey   d. lacrosse

___9. In addition to preventing injuries to the oral cavity, mouthguards also can prevent all but which of the following injuries:
    a. maxillary fractures   c. nasal fractures
    b. temporomandibular joint injuries   d. cerebral concussions

___10. Standards for eye protectors are established by the:
    a. ASTM   c. NCAA
    b. NOCSAE   d. HECC

___11. The best protection from eye injury is:
    a. wearing soft contact lenses   c. wearing open eye guards
    b. wearing polycarbonate eye frames   d. wearing glass lenses

___12. Cervical collars or neck rolls are used to:
    a. decrease axial loading   c. decrease hyperflexion
    b. decrease risk of burners   d. decrease concussions

_13. Quarterbacks and receivers often use the _____type of shoulder pads.
    a. low impact   c. flat
    b. high resilient   d. cantilevered
_14. In football, the greatest amount of force extended on the shoulder region occurs on the ____.
    a. clavicle   c. scapula
    b. acromion process   d. humerus
_15. To determine a player's chest size, circumference measurements should be made:
    a. at the nipple line   c. at the xyphoid process
    b. at the axillary line   d. with arms above the head
_16. The ___ is often used with tennis elbow to reduce tensile forces in the wrist extensors.
    a. neoprene sleeve   c. counterforce forearm band
    b. counterforce humeral band   d. supinator support sleeve
_17. Neoprene sleeves are used for all but which of the following?
    a. provide uniform compression   c. provide stability for a joint injury
    b. provide moderate support for a   d. provide therapeutic warmth
       muscular injury
_18. Functional knee braces are widely used for injuries to the_____.
    a. medial collateral ligament   c. posterior cruciate ligament
    b. lateral collateral ligament   d. anterior cruciate ligament
_19. Use of braces in the treatment of recurring patellofemoral subluxation or dislocation has been found to relieve pain and tension on the ____.
    a. quadricep extension mechanism   c. pes anserine insertion
    b. quadricep flexion mechanism   d. patella tendon
_20. ____ankle braces are more effective than other braces in reducing the frequency of ankle injuries.
    a. lace-up   c. air bladder
    b. semirigid   d. air bladder and semirigid

V. Additional Activities

1. **Practice properly fitting football helmets according to Field Strategy 6-1 on page 186 in the text.**

2. **Practice properly fitting shoulder pads according to Field Strategy 6-3 on page 194 in the text.**

3. **Visit a dentist and have the dentist demonstrate how custom-made mouthguards are made.**

4. **Practice properly fitting mouth-formed mouthguards according to Field Strategy 6-2 on page 190 in the text.**

5. **Visit with the equipment manager at your school and have the manager demonstrate the proper fitting of various types of equipment for different sports.**

6. **Visit an athletic shoe store and ask the salesperson to discuss the various types of running shoes and how the shoes are fitted to different types of feet and running styles.**

I. Key Terms

In vivo — — — — — — — Occurring within the living organism or body

Prophylactic — — — — — To prevent or protect

Diffuse injury — — — — — Injury over a large body area, usually due to low-velocity, high-mass forces

Focal injury — — — — — Injury over a small concentrated area, usually due to high-velocity, low-mass forces

Resilience — — — — — — The ability to bounce or spring back into shape or position after being stretched, bent, or impacted

High-density material — — Materials that absorb more energy from higher impact intensity levels through deformation, thus transferring less stress to a body part

Low-density material — — Materials that absorb energy from low impact intensity levels

II. Simulations

 High Velocity-Low Mass Force

Refer to Table 6-1 on page 184 in the text

Did you suspect the pitcher sustained a thigh contusion? This type of injury is considered to be a focal injury. Did you determine that the force produced by the baseball was one of high-velocity and low mass?

1A. Did you treat the injury by applying the PRICE principle? Did you choose to use padding that was nonresilient and made of high-density material such as orthoplast or thermoplast? Did you layer the padding by using a soft lower density material covered by a firmer higher density material to better absorb and disperse higher intensity blows?

(Refer to Field Strategy 6-2 on page 190 in the text)

Did you suggest that a properly fitted mouthguard can:
- absorb energy
- disperse impact
- cushion the contact between the upper and lower teeth
- keep the upper lip away from the incisal edges of teeth which all significantly reduces dental and oral soft tissue injuries, and to a lesser extent, jaw fractures, cerebral concussion, and temporomandibular joint injuries.

2A. Did you purchase mouthguards that are:
- durable
- resilient
- resistant to tear
- inexpensive
- easy to fabricate
- tasteless and odorless
- clearly visible to officials

Did you use the following guidelines to fit the mouthguards?
- submerge the mouthguard in boiling water for 20 to 25 seconds or until pliable
- shake off excess water but do not rinse in cold water
- place the mouthguard directly in the mouth over the upper dental arch and center it by using the thumbs
- close the mouth but do not bring the teeth together or bite down on the mouthguard.
- instruct the athlete to place the tongue on the roof of the mouth and suck as hard as possible for 15 to 25 seconds
- remove the mouthguard and rinse in cold water to harden the material
- check the mouthguard for any significant indentations on the bottom surface to ensure it is centered correctly

III. Situations

l. Fitting of Football Helmets - (Refer to Field Strategy 6-1 on page 186 in the text) - Did you use the following guidelines to fit the football helmet?

- hair should be cut and wet
- helmet should fit snugly around all of the player's head with cheek pads snug against the sides of the face
- helmet should set 3/4 inch above the player's eyebrows
- face mask should extend two finger widths away from the forehead
- face mask should allow for complete field of vision
- back of helmet should cover the base of the skull
- the ear holes should match up with external auditory ear canal
- chin strap should fit securely
- the helmet should not move when the face guard is pulled up and down or side to side
- the warning label must be on all helmets and clearly visible

2. Fitting of Shoulder Pads - (Refer to Field Strategy 6-3 on page 194 in the text) - Did you use the following guidelines to fit the shoulder pads?

- determine the player's chest size by measuring the circumference of the nipple line
- place the pads on the shoulders
- the straps should be snug enough to prevent no more than a two finger width distance between the pads and body
- the entire clavicle should be covered and protected by the pads
- the acromioclavicular joint should be adequately covered and protected by the upper portion of the arch and deltoid padding
- the entire deltoid should be adequately covered and protected by the extension arch padding
- the entire scapula should be covered with the lower pad arch extending below the inferior angle of the scapula
- with the arms abducted, the neck opening should not be uncomfortable or pinch the neck

3. Bicycle Helmet - (Refer to Figure 6-2 on page 186 in the text) - Did you advise the cyclist to purchase a plastic or fiberglass rigid shell helmet with a chin strap and energy-absorbing foam liner that fits snugly?

4. Eye Protector - Did you suggest an eye protector that:

- is made of polycarbonate
- has a frame constructed of resilient plastic with reinforced temples, hinges, and nose piece
- has adequate cushioning to protect the eyebrows and nasal bridge
- has 3-mm thick lenses
- meet the standards of the American Society for Testing Materials

5. Contact Lenses -Did you suggest that the swimmer not swim with contact lenses but should wear goggles because of the following:
- pool water causes the contact lens to adhere to the cornea, which reduces the risk of losing the contact lens, but also increases the risk of a corneal infection
- goggles protect against organisms in the water and irritation from the chlorine

If the swimmer insists on wearing the contacts, make sure he/she uses goggles and give instructions to:
- wait 20 to 30 minutes after leaving the water to remove the contacts
- immediately disinfect the contacts once removed

6. Sport Bra - Did you suggest the following when purchasing a sport bra?
- it should have no irritative seams or fasteners next to the skin
- it should have nonslip straps
- it should be firm and durable
- it should be a cotton/poly/lycra fabric

7. Functional Knee Brace - Did you determine that a derotational brace be worn by the softball player? The derotational brace is designed to control tibial translation and rotational stress relative to the femur, with a rigid snug fit, and extension limitations?

8. Shin guards - Did you determine that since the force produced by a kick to the shin or a soccer ball to the shin is a high-velocity, low-mass force, the material used for the shin guards should be of high-density padding covered by a molded hard shell?

9. External Ankle Support - Did you determine that the baseball player could benefit from an external ankle supportive device, such as a lace-up, semirigid, or air bladder model? These devices are easy to apply by the wearer, do not irritate the skin as much, provide better comfort and fit, and are more cost-effective. Yes, the use of an external supportive device should be used in combination with a full rehabilitation program to strengthen the muscles around the ankle joint.

10. Athletic Shoes - (Refer to Field Strategy 6-4 on page 209 in the text) - Did the you suggest the following when purchasing athletic shoes for the woman tennis player with high arches?
- use retailers that employ a professional shoe fitter or someone who knows about biomechanics and foot problems
- always fit shoes toward late afternoon or evening to accommodate for any increase in size from the start of the day

III. Situations (Con't)

10. Athletic Shoes (Con't)
- wear socks typically worn during sport participation
- fit shoes to the longest toe of the larger foot
- the shoe should provide one thumb's width from the longest toe to the end of the shoe box
- with both shoes on, approximate athletic skills in the shoes
- the widest part of the shoe should coincide with the widest part of the foot
- women with larger or wider feet should consider purchasing boys' or men's shoes
- court shoes such as those worn for tennis need more side-to-side stability
- individuals with high arches may prefer shoes with soft midsoles, curved lasts, and low or moderate hindfoot stability
- after purchasing the shoes, walk in them for 2 to 3 days to allow them to adapt to the feet and begin using the shoes for activity for about 25 to 30% of the workout, to gradually extending the length of the time the shoes are worn

IV. Multiple Choice Answers

1. b	8. a	15. a
2. a	9. c	16. c
3. b	10. a	17. c
4. c	11. b	18. d
5. c	12. b	19. a
6. d	13. d	20. d
7. b	14. b	

Chapter 7 — The Foot, Ankle and Leg

After completing this chapter you should be able to:

- Locate the bony and soft tissue structures of the foot, ankle, and the lower leg

- Analyze the function of the plantar arches and their role in supporting and distributing body weight

- Describe the motions of the foot and ankle and identify the muscles that produce them

- Explain what forces produce the loading patterns responsible for common injuries to the foot, ankle, and lower leg

- Identify basic principles for preventing injuries to the foot, ankle, and lower leg

- Recognize and manage specific injuries of the foot, ankle, and lower leg

- Demonstrate a thorough assessment of the foot, ankle, and lower leg

- Demonstrate general rehabilitation exercises for the region

I. Anatomy Review

Materials Needed:

SKELETON   ANATOMICAL FOOT/ANKLE/LOW LEG CHARTS   NONPERMANENT MARKERS

Instructions: *Work with a partner to perform the following:*
  - identify the following anatomic structures on the skeleton or anatomical charts
  - palpate and draw the anatomic structures on your partner using the non-permanent marker.

Structures of the Foot

- fourteen phalanges
- distal interphalangeal joint
- proximal interphalangeal joint
- extensor hallucis longus
- flexor hallucis longus and brevis
- extensor digitorum longus
- flexor digitorum longus
- five metatarsal bones

- metatarsophalangeal joint
- head of first metatarsal
- styloid process of fifth metatarsal
- navicular
- cuboid
- three cuneiform bones
- intermetatarsal joint
- tarsometatarsal joint

Structures of the Foot (Con't)

-calcaneus
-longitudinal arch
-transverse arch
-metatarsal arch
-spring ligament or plantar calcaneonavicular
 ligament
-long plantar ligament

-short plantar ligament
-plantar fascia or plantar aponeurosis
-posterior tibialis
-anterior tibialis
-peroneal longus
-peroneal brevis

Structures of the Ankle

-talus
-medial malleolus
-lateral malleolus
-subtalar joint or talocalcaneal joint
-talocrural joint
-deltoid ligament

-anterior talofibular ligament
-calcanealfibular ligament
-posterior talofibular ligament
-Achilles tendon
-retrocalcaneal bursa
-calcaneal bursa

Structures of the Lower Leg

-shaft of the tibia
-distal tibiofibular joint (syndesmosis)
-interosseus membrane
-anterior tibial artery or dorsalis pedis artery
-posterior tibial artery
-tibial nerve
-anterior compartment
-lateral compartment
-superficial posterior compartment
-deep posterior compartment

-gastrocnemius
-soleus
-plantaris
-peroneal longus
-peroneal brevis
-anterior tibialis
-posterior tibialis
-head of fibula
-common peroneal nerve

II. Key Terms

Instructions: *On a separate sheet of paper define the following terms.*

Plantar flexion
Dorsiflexion
Inversion
Eversion
Pronation
Supination
Hallux
Plantar fascia
Metatarsalgia
Pes planus
Pes cavus
Kinetics
Kinematics

Amenorrhea
Osteopenia
Oligomenorrhea
Paronychia
Hammer toes
Claw toes
Keratolytic agent
Tinea pedis
Verrucae plantaris
Stratum corneum
Neuritis
Freiberg's disease
Heel bruise

Sever's disease
Shin bruise
Syndesmosis
Tenosynovitis
Snowball crepitation
Bimalleolar fracture
Jones fracture
Nonunion fracture
Osteochondritis dissecans
Compartment syndrome
Chronic exertional
  compartment syndrome

III. Kinematics of the Foot, Ankle, and Lower Leg

Instructions: *Work with a partner to perform the following. Have your partner perform the following movements while you name the muscles that are performing the movements along with the normal range of motion for each movement.*

The injured athlete should perform the following movements. The athletic trainer should name the muscles performing the motion and provide the normal range of motion for each movement. (Refer to pages 223–232 and 259–260 in text)

	Muscle	**Range of Motion**
-flexion of the second to fifth toes		
-flexion of the first toe		
-extension of the first toe		
-dorsiflexion		
-plantar flexion		
-inversion		
-eversion		

After you have determined range of motion by subjective measures, determine both dorsiflexion and plantar flexion using a goniometer.

IV. Simulations

Instructions: *Perform the following simulations.*
A cross-country runner reports to the training room complaining of pain along the plantar surface of the left foot. Complete a history and observation for this injury.

1A. After completing the history, you have found the runner has been increasing his distance and has been running more frequently on street-like surfaces. He has more pain in the morning when he awakes, and then the pain diminishes. After he runs, the pain returns. His shoes are somewhat old and worn. He has some pes planus on the left foot when compared to the right foot. There is minor swelling along the longitudinal medial border but no discoloration. Continue the palpation and special testing procedures.

1B. After palpation and special testing, you find pinpoint pain near the superior medial aspect of the calcaneus and along the medial longitudinal arch. Increased pain was present on active and resistive toe flexion. Pain also increased with passive extension of the toes and dorsiflexion of the ankle. What type of condition do you suspect? What treatment do you recommend?

A guard on the basketball team went down on the court holding her ankle. After being beckoned onto the court, you find the guard injured her right ankle through a plantar flexion inversion force. She had no previous injury to this ankle. Perform an on-the-court evaluation and demonstrate how to move the guard from the court to the sidelines.

2A. The athlete is now on the sidelines. Perform a more in-depth palpation and special testing portion of the assessment.

2B. What criteria will determine if the guard can reenter the game? Demonstrate the functional testing the athlete should be able to perform prior to reentering the game. Will any type of protective strapping, bracing, or taping be used? If yes, which technique will be used and why? Demonstrate its application. What treatment do you recommend?

A middle-aged tennis player was playing on a cool day when the individual felt a sudden, painful tearing sensation in the calf, leading to immediate disability. What factors may have contributed to this injury? Perform the observation and palpation procedures for this injury. During the assessment, differentiate between bone and soft tissue injury.

3A. After performing the observation and palpation, you find the area is swollen, point tender, discolored, and the athlete is experiencing muscle spasms. Continue with special testing.

3B. After performing range of motion and other special testing procedures, you find the athlete unable to bear weight and actively plantar flex the affected foot. What injury should be suspected? What is the immediate treatment protocol?

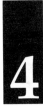

During preseason conditioning a volleyball player developed pain along the distal medial tibial border that is present at the start of practice and running. The pain diminishes as activity progresses only to recur after activity ends. What factors may initiate this condition? How will you determine the difference between bone and soft tissue injury? Perform observation and palpation procedures for this injury?

4A. After performing observation and palpation, you find the athlete has noticeable foot pronation on the affected leg and pes planus. The area is point tender but not swollen, hot, or discolored. The athlete has a dorsal pedis pulse and has normal sensory function. What injury should be suspected? How should this injury be managed?

V. Situations

<u>Instructions:</u> *Work with a partner to cooperatively analyze and address the following situations.*

l. A defensive back has throbbing pain on the plantar side of the great toe on the right foot. The pain increases significantly when the athlete pushes off the right foot to block an opponent. What might have caused this condition? What injury should be suspected? Demonstrate the treatment protocol for this injury.

2. A basketball player has an aggravating pain in the Achilles tendon region of the left lower leg. This pain has been present for the past 2 weeks. Determine the difference between tendon and bursa injury. Determine the severity of this injury. How should this injury be managed?

3. A field hockey player's foot was stepped on by an opposing player. Demonstrate how a possible fracture to the metatarsals and phalanges should be determined. Should sensation and circulation be checked? If yes, demonstrate these procedures.

4. After wrestling practice, a wrestler complains of a dry itching sensation on his feet and between his toes. Observation reveals dry vesicular lesions and cracking fissures of the skin. What factors may produce these signs and symptoms? What condition should be suspected? How should this condition be managed?

5. A soccer player was hit on the left superior lateral leg. Although the initial pain subsided, the dorsum of the foot feels somewhat numb. Determine the difference between a contusion and an acute compartment syndrome. What complications might occur from this type of injury? What should the immediate treatment be for this injury?

6. A basketball player is recovering from a mild, second-degree inversion ankle sprain. After controlling acute swelling and inflammation, what exercises should be included in the rehabilitation program?

VI. Special Tests

<u>Instructions:</u> *Work with a partner to perform and explain the rationale for each of the following special tests.*

-Thompson test   -Anterior drawer test   -Talar tilt

VII. Multiple Choice Questions

Instructions: Choose the best answer for each question.

___1.   The closed packed position of the tarsometatarsal and intermetatarsal joints is:
a. plantar flexion   c. supination
b. dorsiflexion   d. pronation

___2.   The ____ joint is considered the true ankle joint.
a. subtalar   c. talocalcaneonavicular
b. talocrural   d. transverse

___3.   Forces producing stress on the medial aspect of the ankle typically cause:
a. tearing of the deltoid ligament
b. syndesmosis sprain
c. stress fracture of the medial malleolus
d. avulsion fracture of the medial malleolus

___4.   The ____ ligament is the primary supporter of the medial longitudinal arch.
a. long plantar   c. calcaneonavicular
b. short plantar   d. interosseous tibiofibular

___5.   Inversion and eversion movements primarily occur at the:
a. talocrural joint   c. tarsometatarsal joints
b. intertarsal joints   d. subtalar joint

___6.   Excessive____ is often associated with Achilles tendon stress, plantar fasciitis, and medial tibial stress syndrome.
a. inversion   c. pronation
b. eversion   d. supination

___7.   To increase strength of the plantar surface of the foot, an athlete could:
a. perform toe flexion exercises
b. perform toe extension exercises
c. perform bilateral heel raises
d. perform inversion and eversion exercises

___8.   All of the following are recommendations in preventing tinea pedis but:
a. drying feet thoroughly after showers
b. wearing no socks during exercise
c. applying an absorbent powder to the feet
d. clean and disinfect shower room floors

___9.   Compression of the medial and lateral plantar nerves of the metatarsal heads can lead to _____.
a. plantar fasciitis   c. Freiberg's disease
b. metatarsalgia   d. plantars' neuroma

___10.   Palpable pain in the soft tissue just anterior to the Achilles tendon in a runner can be indicative of_____.
a. retrocalcaneal bursitis   c. Achilles tendinitis
b. posterior calcaneal bursitis   d. an exostosis

___11.   When applying ice to a contusion to the gastrocnemius, the muscle should be _____ to decrease muscle spasms.
a. kept in dorsiflexion   c. in a relaxed position
b. kept in plantar flexion   d. left alone

___12. Acute anterior compartment syndrome may occur do to all the following but:
a. direct blow
b. fracture
c. shin splints
d. circulatory occlusion

___13. Immediate care of acute anterior compartment syndrome involves all of the following but:
a. physician referral
b. ice or cold applications
c. rest
d. compression

___14. Individuals with _____ are at risk for medial ankle sprains.
a. supination
b. pronation
c. pes cavus
d. tight Achilles tendons

___15. Snowball crepitation is associated with_____.
a. bony fractures
b. tendinitis
c. tenosynovitis
d. bursitis

___16. _____dislocations can be overlooked or confused with an ankle sprain because it also gives a feeling of instability and pain over the lateral malleolus.
a. subtalar joint
b. peroneal tendon
c. syndesmosis
d. tibialis posterior tendon

___17. The _____ test is used to determine Achilles tendon rupture.
a. talar tilt
b. Thomas
c. anterior drawer
d. Thompson

___18. Pain along the medial tibial border that diminishes as activity progresses and returns hours after activity has ceased may be indicative of_____.
a. medial tibial stress syndrome
b. tibialis posterior tendinitis
c. exercise-induced compartment syndrome
d. tibial stress fracture

___19. In chronic anterior compartment syndrome, _____ is weak and limited.
a. plantar flexion
b. dorsiflexion
c. inversion
d. eversion

___20. Palpable heel pain just below the Achilles tendon attachment that increases with activity and diminishes with rest in the adolescent aged 10 to 15 may be indicative of:
a. Achilles tendinitis
b. heel bruise
c. retrocalcaneal bursitis
d. apophysitis of the calcaneus

VIII. Additional Activities

1. Visit a radiologist at a nearby hospital and ask the radiologist to share various x-rays of the foot and ankle with you to view various foot structures.

2. Visit a podiatrist and have the podiatrist share with you the various types of orthotics used for various foot structures and foot injuries.

3. Design a rehabilitation program for an athlete suffering from an acute lateral ankle sprain.

4. Design a rehabilitation program for an athlete suffering from plantar fasciitis.

I. Anatomy

Refer to Table 7-1 on page 228 in the text

II. Key Terms

Hallux — — — — — — — The first or great toe

Plantar fascia — — — — — Specialized band of fascia that covers the plantar surface of the foot and helps support the longitudinal arch

Metatarsalgia — — — — — A condition involving general discomfort around the metatarsal heads

Pes planus — — — — — — Flat feet

Pes cavus — — — — — — High arches

Pronation — — — — — — Combined motions of calcaneal eversion, foot abduction, and dorsiflexion

Supination — — — — — — Combined motions of calcaneal inversion, foot adduction, and plantar flexion

Kinetics — — — — — — — Study of the forces causing and resulting from motion

Kinematics — — — — — — Study of the spatial and temporal aspects of movement

Amenorrhea — — — — — Absence or abnormal stoppage of menses

Osteopenia — — — — — — Pathological condition of reduced bone mineral density

Oligomenorrhea — — — — Menstruation involving scant blood loss

Paronychia — — — — — — A fungal/bacterial infection in the folds of the skin surrounding a fingernail or toenail

Hammer toes — — — — — A flexion deformity of the distal interphalangeal (DIP) joint of the toes

Claw toes — — — — — — A toe deformity characterized by hyperextension of the metatarsophalangeal (MP) joint and hyperflexion of the interphalangeal (IP) joint

II. Key Terms (Con't)

Keratolytic agent — — —   An agent that promotes softening and dissolution or peeling of the horny layer of skin

Tinea pedis — — — — —   A common fungal infection found between the toes characterized by small vesicles, itching, and scaling

Verrucae plantaris — — —   Plantars' warts

Stratum corneum — — —   The outermost layer of the epidermis; horny layer of cells that are dead

Neuritis — — — — — —   Inflammation or irritation of a nerve commonly found between the third and fourth metatarsal heads

Freiberg's disease — — —   Avascular necrosis that occurs to the second metatarsal head in some adolescents

Heel bruise — — — — —   Contusion to the subcutaneous fat pad located over the inferior aspect of the calcaneus

Sever's disease — — — —   A traction-type injury, or osteochondrosis, of the calcaneal apophysis seen in young adolescents

Shin bruise — — — — —   A contusion of the tibia, sometimes referred to as tibial periostitis

Syndesmosis — — — — —   A joint where the opposing surfaces are joined together by fibrous connective tissue

Tenosynovitis — — — — —   Inflammation of the inner lining of the tendon sheath caused by friction between the tendon and the sheath

Snowball crepitation — —   Sound similar to that heard when crunching snow into a snowball, indicating presence of tenosynovitis

Bimalleolar fracture — —   Fractures of both the medial and lateral malleolus

Bipartite — — — — — —   Having two parts

Jones Fracture — — — —   A transverse stress fracture of the proximal shaft of the fifth metatarsal

Nonunion fracture — — —   A fracture where healing is delayed or fails to unite at all

II. Key Terms (Con't)

Osteochondritis dissecans — Inflammation of both bone and cartilage that can split the pieces into the joint, resulting in loss of blood supply to the fragments

Compartment syndrome —— A condition where increased intramuscular pressure is brought on by activity that impedes blood flow and function of tissues within that compartment

Chronic exertional — — — Intermittent excessive pressure that reduces blood flow compartment syndrome through a muscular compartment causing pain and possible paresthesia

III. Kinematics of the Foot, Ankle, and Lower Leg

Movement	Muscles	Normal ROM
Flexion of second to fifth toes	Flexor digitorum longus	
Flexion of first toe	Flexor hallucis longus	
Extension of first toe	Extensor hallucis longus	
Dorsi flexion	Extensor hallucis longus	20°
	Anterior tibialis	
	Extensor digitorum longus	
Plantar flexion	Gastrocnemius	30°–50°
	Soleus	
	Plantaris	
Supination	Tibialis posterior	45°– 60°
	Tibialis anterior	
Pronation	Peroneals	15° –30°

Refer to Table 7-1 on page 228 and pages 259 to 260 in the text.

IV. Simulations

 Plantar fasciitis

During the history did you:
- determine if the injury was chronic or acute
- ask questions about training regimen (time, distance, surface, progression)
- ask questions about type of shoes
- ask where, when, how the injury occurred
- ask about previous injury, treatment, or medications
- ask about the type of pain the athlete is experiencing (dull, sharp, radiating, constant, intermittent, localized, general, increased during activity)
- ask if rest helped the injury

Plantar fasciitis (Con't)

1A. Did you palpate the following structures for point tenderness, swelling, deformity, sensation, or other signs of trauma?
-metatarsal arch
-transverse arch
-longitudinal arch
-calcaneous
-plantar surface of foot

During the special tests did you:
- perform the squeeze test for possible stress fracture of metatarsals
- have the athlete flex and extend toes as well as plantar flex and dorsiflex the ankle
- stretch the plantar surface of the foot by having the athlete extend the toes while passively dorsiflexing the foot
- apply resistance to toe flexion
- have the athlete walk, run, or perform other functional activities

1B. Did you suspect plantar fasciitis?
(Refer to Field Strategy 7-5 on text page 249 for management of fasciitis)

2 **Ankle Sprain**

During the court evaluation did you:
-ask why, how, and what questions
-ask questions concerning location and severity of pain
-ask about previous injury
-observe the region around the ankle with the shoe on for swelling, discoloration, or deformity
-perform special testing for fractures with the shoe on
-ask the athlete to move the ankle with the shoe on after performing a negative stress test for fracture
-remove the athlete from the court with an assistive or nonassistive carrying mode depending on the extent of injury

2A. After the athlete was assisted to the sidelines and the shoe and sock were removed, did you palpate the following structures for swelling, deformity, and point tenderness?

-metatasals
-tarsal bones
-medial and lateral malleolus
-sinus tarsi area and anterior talofibular ligament
-calcaneofibular ligament
-posterior talofibular ligament
-deltoid ligament
-Achilles tendon
-calcaneus
-palpate bilaterally

Did you perform the following special tests?

-range of motion (passive, active, and resistive)
-stress tests for ankle and forefoot fracture
-anterior drawer test and talar tilt
-functional activities (walking, running, jumping)

2B. In determining if the athlete could return to participation, did you rule out:

-fracture
-ligament instability
-dislocation

Did you determine that the athlete could return to participation if the following could be performed without a limp and with very mild discomfort:

-walk, run, jump
-functional activities

Did you use a closed basketweave taping procedure before returning the athlete to the game? After the game, did you apply ICE? (Refer to Field Strategy 7-4 on page 245 in the text for management of lateral ankle sprains)

Did you determine that the following factors may have contributed to the tennis player's injury?
> -lack of flexibility
> -lack of warm-up before activity
> -lack of strength
> -age of athlete
> -overloading mechanism

Did you observe bilaterally for:
> -swelling, discoloration, deformity, other signs of trauma

Did you palpate bilaterally for:
> -swelling, deformity, crepitation, point tenderness, other signs of trauma

Did you determine that bone injuries would have point tenderness over the injury site and possibly a visible deformity, whereas soft tissue injuries would result in more general pain?

3A. During the special tests did you:
> -perform active, passive, and resistive range of motion (if possible)
> -perform stress test for bone fracture of the lower leg
> -perform the Thompson test for Achilles tendon rupture
> -ask the athlete if he or she could bear weight

Did you suspect an Achilles tendon rupture? Did you apply ICE, immobilize, and refer immediately to a physician?

 Medial Tibial Stress Syndrome

Did you determine the following factors could have contributed to the volleyball player's injury?
> -lack of flexibility
> -lack of progression in training regimen
> -changing of running and practice surface
> -overuse
> -lack of supportive footwear

*It is difficult to differentiate between bone and soft tissue injury of this area. Treatment of either injury is the same. If the injury does not respond to the treatment, referral to a physician is needed.

Did you observe bilaterally for:
-deformity, swelling, discoloration, other signs of trauma
-posture abnormalities (genu valgus and varus, ankle pronation and supination, tibial torsion, pelvic tilt, short leg syndrome, pes planus, pes cavus)
-the athlete's footwear
-the athlete's walking gait pattern

Did you palpate the following structures bilaterally for swelling, deformity, point tenderness, temperature, and other signs of trauma?
-anterior tibialis
-medial shaft of the tibia
-interosseus membrane
-syndesmosis

Did you palpate for sensation and circulation?

4A. Did you suspect this injury to be medial tibial stress syndrome? (Refer to Field Strategy 7-6 on page 251 in the text for management procedures for medial tibial stress syndrome)

V. Situations

1. Turf Toe - Did you determine this condition to be turf toe? Did you determine that lack of supportive toe counters in the athlete's shoes and playing on turf were factors that may have contributed to this injury? To manage this condition did you:
-apply ICE
-use a turf toe supportive tape procedure or strap for support
-work on range of motion and strength when applicable

2. Achilles Tendonitis - Did you determine that the basketball player was experiencing Achilles tendonitis rather than retrocalcaneal bursitis by palpating the Achilles tendon and retrocalcaneal bursa for:
-point tenderness
-swelling
-deformity
-temperature
-crepitation

V. Situations (Con't)

Did you determine the severity of this injury by looking for functional limitations and points of pain as the athlete performed:
- range of motion: active, passive, resistive
- functional activities, walking, running, jumping, and so forth
- the Thompson test for integrity of the Achilles tendon

Did your treatment protocol include:
- apply ICE
- apply a heel lift for support
- begin range of motion and strength exercises when applicable

3. Metatarsal Fracture - To check for stress fracture of the metarsals and phalanges did you perform the squeeze test, compression, or distraction test? Did you check for sensation and circulation? **Refer to Field Strategy 7-9 on page 259 in the text to determine a possible fracture of the foot and lower leg.**

4. Tinea Pedis - Did you determine that the condition of the wrestler could be tinea pedis? Did you determine that the following conditions could contribute to tinea pedis?
- lack of drying feet after showers
- lack of wearing shoes in showers and locker rooms
- wearing colored socks when feet are wet or in wet footwear
(Refer to Field Strategy 7-3 on page 238 in the text for management of tinea pedis [athlete's foot])

5. Acute Anterior Compartment Syndrome - To differentiate between a contusion or an acute compartment syndrome sustained by the soccer player did you:
- palpate for swelling, deformity, temperature, and other signs of trauma
- check for pulse in the anterior tibial artery and dorsalis pedis artery
- check for sensation

Did you determine the following complications?
- loss of sensation
- decreased functional abnormalities
- diminished pulse
- contusion to the peroneal nerve
- fracture to the fibula

In the treatment protocol did you use ice but not compression because external compression will hasten tissue deterioration? Did you choose not to elevate the limb because of decreased arterial pressure? Did you immediately refer the athlete to a physician?

V. Situations (Con't)

6. Ankle Rehabilitation Exercises - Did you include the following exercises in the rehabilitation plan?
- -ankle alphabet
- -triceps surae stretch
- -theraband or surgical tubing exercises in all ranges of ankle motion
- -unilateral balance exercises
- -BAPS board or other proprioception exercises

(Refer to Field Strategy 7-10 on page 265 in the text)

VI. Special Test

Refer to pages 259 to 264 in the text

VII. Multiple Choice Answers

l. c	8. b	15. c
2. b	9. d	16. b
3. d	10. a	17. d
4. c	11. a	18. a
5. d	12. c	19. b
6. c	13. d	20. d
7. a	14. b	

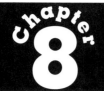

The Knee

After completing this chapter you should be able to:

- Locate the important bony and soft tissue structures of the knee region

- Describe the motions of the knee and identify the muscles that produce them

- Explain what forces produce the loading patterns responsible for common injuries at the knee

- Recognize specific injuries at the knee

- Describe and demonstrate an assessment of the knee and patellofemoral joint

- Identify protective padding and commercial products to assist in the prevention and management of knee and patella injuries

- Demonstrate general rehabilitation exercises for the region

I. Anatomy Review

Materials Needed:

SKELETON   ANATOMICAL KNEE CHARTS   NONPERMANENT MARKERS

Instructions: *Work with a partner to perform the following:*
  - identify the following anatomical structures on the skeleton or anatomical charts
  - palpate and draw the anatomical structures on your partner using the nonpermanent marker.

———————————— Structures of the Knee ————————————

-tibiofemoral joint
-patellofemoral joint
-tibia
-femur
-fibula
-medial and lateral tibial plateaus
-medial and lateral femoral condyles
-head of fibula
-patella
-trochlear groove

-medial meniscus
-lateral meniscus
-suprapatellar bursa
-superficial infrapatellar bursa
-deep infrapatellar bursa
-prepatella bursa
-subpopliteal bursa
-pes anserine bursa
-tibial collateral ligament
-fibular collateral ligament

-anterior cruciate
-posterior cruciate
-coronary ligaments
-meniscofemoral ligament
-arcuate ligament
-popliteal space
-gracilis
-sartorius
-semimembranosus
-semitendinosus
-iliotibial band
-Gerdy's tubercle

-rectus femoris
-vastus lateralis
-vastus medialis
-vastus intermedius
-biceps femoris
-popliteus
-gastrocnemius
-plantaris
-tibial nerve
-common peroneal nerve
-popliteal artery

II. Key Terms

Instructions: *On a separate sheet of paper define the following terms.*

Intracapsular
Extrasynovial
Menisci
Bucket-handle tear
Parrot-beak tear
Collateral ligaments
Valgus laxity
Varus laxity

Cruciate ligaments
Tibiofemoral joint
Patellofemoral joint
Chondromalacia patellae
Patellofemoral stress
  syndrome
Patella plica
Extensor mechanism
Q-angle

Screwing home mechanism
Chondral fracture
Osteochondral fracture
Osteochondritis dissecans
Larsen-Johansson disease
Osgood-Schlatter disease
Arthralgia
Hemarthrosis
Neoplasm

III. Kinematics

Instructions: *Work with a partner to perform the following. Have your partner perform the following movements while you name the muscles that are performing the movements along with the normal range of motion for each movement.*

	Muscle	**Range of Motion**
-knee flexion		
-knee extension		
-medial rotation of the tibia		
-lateral rotation of the tibia		
-patellofemoral joint motion		

After you have determined the range of motion of the knee joint through subjective means, measure both knee flexion and extension with a goniometer.

IV. Simulations

 A distance runner has pain on weight bearing and mild swelling on the anteromedial aspect of the proximal tibia just below the joint line. This injury has been irritating the runner for 2 weeks. Perform a history, observation, and palpation of this injury.

lA. After completing the history of the injury, you learned that the runner's training mileage has significantly increased during the past 3 weeks, although intensity has remained the same. However, it now hurts the runner just to walk. Observation reveals minor swelling over the area and moderate pronation and pes planus on the affected leg. The shoes are worn but still in adequate shape for the training required. Palpation reveals point tenderness over the medial tibial plateau. What condition do you suspect and how will you manage this injury?

 A field hockey player was hit on the anterolateral side of the proximal tibia of the left shin with an opposing player's stick. Swelling occurred rapidly, but there is no discoloration or deformity noted during the observation. Perform palpation and stress testing procedures.

2A. Palpation reveals point tenderness over the proximal tibia area. The player has some loss of sensation distal to the injury, but the individual has full movement capabilities and a strong dorsalis pedis pulse. What is your management plan? What signs would indicate immediate referral to a physician is necessary?

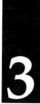 **A basketball player decelerated, set the left foot, then forcefully pushed off the left leg to perform a righthanded layup shot. However, the player suddenly fell to the floor, grasping the left knee. The individual reported a popping sensation and a feeling of giving way in the knee. Extreme pain is evident over the anteromedial joint line. Explain and demonstrate your on-the-court evaluation for this injury.**

3A. Within minutes, rapid joint effusion and tenderness are present over the anteromedial joint line and in the posterior aspect of the knee. When performing the Lachman test, pain increased and some instability was present. How would you remove the athlete from the court? Explain and demonstrate your off-the-court evaluation.

3B. After completing the off-the-court evaluation you found a positive Lachman test and positive valgus stress test. The individual has limited flexion and extension due to joint effusion. What structures at the knee may be injured and how would you manage this injury?

A young hockey player is complaining of an aching pain in the right knee that begins shortly after the start of practice that just doesn't feel right. Joint effusion and point tenderness over the femoral condyles is apparent after practice, but no history of an actual injury can be recalled. Explain and demonstrate what stress testing procedures should be used with this injury.

4A. The skater has pain in a short arc of motion during resisted knee extension and internal rotation, but not with knee extension and external rotation. You have also found momentary locking of the knee during active knee range of motion. What injury do you suspect and how would you manage this injury?

A female distance runner is complaining of a deep, aching pain in the knee during activity. Explain and demonstrate your history and observation for this chronic injury.

5A. The runner cannot recall any injury to her knee. She has increased her running distance from 4 miles/day to 6 miles/day in the past week and has been running on varied surfaces. Pain is also present during ascending and descending stairs. After practice, she has been applying ice to her knee and taking ibuprofen. Observation reveals no postural abnormalities other than a moderate patella alta, and slight joint effusion. Explain and demonstrate your palpation and stress testing procedures.

5B. During palpation of the patella, the athlete reported pain and tenderness when you pushed downward into the patellofemoral groove. She also reports discomfort when moving the patella medially and laterally. During passive knee extension, the patella laterally deviates from the groove. Pain increases during resisted knee extension, and crepitation occurs under the patella. She cannot perform a duck walk or squat test without pain, and has a positive Waldron's test. What condition do you suspect? What factors may have contributed to this type of injury?

V. Situations

Instructions: *Work with a partner to cooperatively analyze and answer the following situations.*

1. A wrestler has a history of a chronic aching, warm, swollen knee. There is no visible patella outline. Do you think the swelling is intraarticular or extraarticular? What is your management plan?

2. A female runner is complaining of an aching sensation on the lateral side of her knee that first began in her hip a week ago. Her pain increases in intensity as milage increases, when running hills, and when going up and down stairs. She also has a feeling of tightness within her knee during knee flexion. What injury do you suspect? What predisposing factors may have contributed to this injury?

3. After performing a history, observation, and palpation on a softball player's acutely injured knee, you have ruled out collateral or cruciate ligament injury. However, you still suspect medial menisci injury. Explain and demonstrate the special tests for medial menisci injury. What constitutes a positive test? Why?

4. A female soccer player was decelerating after a drive to the goal and was cutting upfield to chase an opposing player. Her knee collapses, and she falls to the ground. Observation reveals that the athlete's patella is laterally displaced. How would you manage this injury? Other than the patella, what other structures could be injured?

5. An adolescent basketball player is complaining of bilateral distal patella tendon pain. Explain and demonstrate how you would determine the difference between patella tendinitis and Osgood-Schlatter syndrome. What are the treatment protocols for each condition?

6. After a second degree medial collateral knee injury, an individual is ready to begin active exercise as part of a rehabilitation program. List the types of exercises you would have the individual perform in a nonweight-bearing position.

VI. Special Tests

Instructions: *Work with a partner to perform the following special tests and explain the rational for each test.*

- Lachman
- Anterior drawer
- Posterior drawer
- Valgus and varus stress
- Gravity test
- McMurry's

- Apley compression
- Brush or stroke test
- Ballotable patella
- Patella compression or grind test
- Patella apprehension test
- Ober's test
- Nobel's compression

VII. Multiple Choice Questions

Instructions: Choose the best answer for each question.

___1. All but which of the following are intracapsular structures of the knee?
   a. anterior cruciate ligament   c. medial collateral ligament
   b. posterior cruciate ligament   d. medial menisci

___2. The synovial fluid of the knee is under the least amount of pressure during _____.
   a. full flexion   c. full extension
   b. semiflexion   d. tibial rotation

___3. The _____ nerve courses down the anterior aspect of the thigh.
   a. femoral   c. sciatic
   b. tibial   d. peroneal

___4. Rotational capability of the tibia with respect to the femur is maximal at approximately _____ of knee _____.
   a. 90 degrees, extension   c. 30 degrees, flexion
   b. 90 degrees, flexion   d. 60 degrees, extension

___5. The ___ of the knee acts as the major shock absorbency structure and bears as much as 45% of the total load.
   a. patella   c. meniscus
   b. articular cartilage   d. anterior cruciate ligament

___6. An athlete has received a blow to the anterior lateral lower leg and is experiencing paresthesia along the lateral malleolus. What structure may have been injured?
   a. sciatic nerve   c. peroneal brevis muscle
   b. peroneal nerve   d. posterior compartment

___7. Knee extension and knee flexion exercises are all considered _____ exercises for the knee.
   a. isometric   c. closed chain
   b. static   d. open chain

___8. Bursa about the knee are most commonly injured from _____ forces.
   a. shearing   c. tension
   b. rotational   d. compressive

___9. _____ bursitis is often associated with running and cycling and is routinely aggravated by knee flexion

a. infrapatella
b. deep infrapatella
c. pes Anserine
d. suprapatellar

___10. Ligamentous injuries of the knee are classified by all but which of the following?

a. the degree of laxity
b. the degree of swelling
c. the direction of laxity
d. the functional disruption of the ligament

___11. Anteromedial instability involves injury to all of the following structures except the _____.

a. fibular collateral ligament
b. tibial collateral ligament
c. anterior cruciate ligament
d. medial menisci

___12. Immediate swelling of the knee after acute injury usually indicates _____.

a. fibular collateral injury
b. interarticular joint injury
c. extra-articular joint injury
d. quadriceps mechanism injury

___13. All but which of the following tests are used to identify a menisci injury?

a. McMurray's test
b. Apley compression test
c. duck walk test
d. Lachman test

___14. Atrophy of the _____ is nearly always evident in patella femoral dysfunction.

a. vastus lateralis
b. rectus femoris
c. vastus medialis oblique
d. sartorius

___15. The McConnell taping technique is used to _____.

a. correct patellar position and tracking during knee extension
b. support the popliteal muscle during knee hyperextension
c. support the popliteal space during Baker's cyst formation
d. support the patella tendon during jumper's knee

___16. A popping or snapping sensation during knee flexion with pseudolocking mimicking a menisci injury may be indicative of an injury to the _____.

a. patella tendon
b. insertion of the iliotibial band
c. patella plica
d. quadriceps tendon

___17. Osgood-Schlatter disease is a _____ injury to the tibial apophysis.

a. shearing-like
b. compression
c. traction-like
d. degenerative-like

___18. A runner reports to you with lateral leg pain that is point tender over the femoral condyle about 2 to 3 cm above the lateral joint line. The pain occasionally radiates distally to the tibial attachment or proximally up the thigh. What structure could be involved with this injury?

a. pes anserine tendon
b. iliotibial band
c. rectus femoris
d. fibular collateral ligament

___19. An athlete has received a blow to the anterior knee and has diffused extra-articular swelling and cannot perform a straight leg raise. What injury do you suspect?

a. anterior cruciate tear
b. posterior cruciate tear
c. patella fracture
d. popliteal bursitis

_20.   When observing the knee during injury evaluation, the knee should be in a
position of _____ in order to relieve any strain on the joint structures.
a. full extension   c. full flexion
b. 90 degrees of flexion   d. 30 degrees of flexion

VIII. Additional Activities ———————————————

l. **Develop a rehabilitation program for an athlete who has patella femoral problems.**

2. **Demonstrate closed chain exercises for the knee.**

3. **Visit a physical therapist or athletic trainer and observe the various type of knee
exercises used during knee rehabilitation.**

4. **Visit an athletic trainer and observe the various types of supportive and protective
devices used for the knee.**

I. Anatomy

Refer to Tables 8-1 on page 273 in the text and 8-2 on page 274 in the text

II. Key Terms

Intracapsular — — — — — Structures found within the articular capsule

Extrasynovial — — — — — Structures found outside of the synovial cavity

Menisci — — — — — — — Fibrocartilage discs within the knee joint that reduce joint stress

Bucket-handle tear — — — Longitudinal meniscal tear of the central segment that can displace into the joint, leading to locking of the knee

Parrot-beak tear — — — — Horizontal meniscal tear typically in the middle segment of the lateral meniscus

Collateral ligaments — — — Major ligaments that cross the medial and lateral aspects of the knee

Valgus laxity — — — — — An opening of the medial side of the joint caused by the distal segment moving laterally

Varus laxity — — — — — — An opening on the lateral side of a joint caused by the distal segment moving medially

Cruciate ligaments — — — Major ligaments that crisscross the knee in the anteroposterior direction

Tibiofemoral joint — — — Dual condyloid joints between the tibial and femoral condyles that function primarily as a modified hinge joint

Patellofemoral joint — — — Gliding joint between the patella and the patellar groove of the femur

Chondromalacia patella — Degenerative condition in the articular cartilage of the patella caused by abnormal compression or shearing forces

Patellofemoral stress — — Condition whereby the lateral retinaculum is tight, or the syndrome vastus medialis oblique is weak, leading to lateral excursion and pressure on the lateral facet of the patella causing a painful condition

II. Key Terms (Con't)

Patella plica — — — — — — A fold in the synovial lining that may cause medial knee pain associated with trauma

Extensor mechanism — — Complex interaction of muscles, ligaments, and tendons that stabilize and provide the motion at the patellofemoral joint

Q-angle — — — — — — Angle between the line of the quadriceps force and the patella tendon

Screwing home mechanism— Rotation of the tibia on the femur during extension that produces an anatomical "locking" of the knee

Chondral fracture — — — Fracture involving the articular cartilage at a joint

Osteochondral fracture — — Fracture involving the articular cartilage and underlying bone

Osteochondritis dissecans— Localized area of avascular necrosis, resulting from complete or incomplete separation of joint cartilage and subchondral bone

Larsen-Johansson disease— Inflammation or partial avulsion of the apex of the patella due to traction forces

Osgood-Schlatter disease— Inflammation or partial avulsion of the tibial apophysis due to traction forces

Arthralgia — — — — — — Severe joint pain

Hemarthrosis — — — — — Collection of blood within a joint or cavity

Neoplasm — — — — — — Tumor that can be benign or malignant

III. Kinematics of the Knee

Motion	Muscles	Range of Motion
Knee flexion	Semitendinosus	0–135°
	Semimembranosus	
	Biceps femoris	
	Sartorius	
	Gracilis	
Knee extension	Rectus femoris	0–15°
	Vastus lateralis	
	Vastus medialis	
	Vastus intermedius	
Medial rotation of the tibia	Sartorius	20–30°
	Semitendinosus	
	Semimembranosus	
	Gracilis	
Lateral rotation of the tibia	Biceps femoris	30–40°
Patellofemoral joint motion	Vastus medialis	

IV. Simulations

 Medial Tibial Plateau Stress Fracture

During the history, did you ask:
- what, when, and how questions
- about past injury, treatment, medications
- type of pain
- changes in training, running surface, distance, mileage
- changes in footwear
- pain during activity or inactivity
- functional abilities

During observation, did you bilaterally observe:
- for swelling, discoloration, deformity, other signs of trauma
- pes planus, pes cavus, foot pronation, foot supination
- genu valgus, varus, tibial torsion
- leg length discrepancies
- walking gait pattern
- shoe wear

During palpation, did you bilaterally palpate for:
- swelling, temperature, deformity, point tenderness, other signs of trauma
- possible fracture

lA. Did you suspect the runner had a stress fracture of the medial tibial plateau? This may be due to the repetitive overuse from the increased mileage. In addition, the point tenderness over the medial tibial plateau should have identified a possible bony injury. Did you include the following in the management plan?
- ice to control pain
- crutch fitting
- physician referral for a radiograph
- rest from weight-bearing activities
- gradual progression back into weight-bearing activities

2 **Contusion**

During palpation, did you bilaterally palpate for:
- swelling, temperature, deformity, crepitation, and other signs of trauma
- possible fracture
- sensory function distal to the injury site
- a distal pulse

During the special tests, did you:
- test for a possible fracture to the head of the fibula and proximal tibia
- test for motor functioning
- test for nerve functioning

2A. During the management plan, did you:
- apply ice, compression, and elevation to the injury
- continue to monitor sensation and pulse

Did you determine that the following would indicate an immediate referral to a physician?
- signs of a possible fracture
- loss of motor functioning
- further loss of sensation
- decreased or lack of pulse

During the on-the-court evaluation, did you:
  Take a quick history by asking:
  - what, when, and how questions
  - previous injury

  Observe bilaterally for:
  - swelling, deformity, discoloration, other signs of trauma

  Palpate for:
  - areas of point tenderness, swelling, deformity, temperature, crepitation, and other signs of trauma
  - a possible fracture

Did you ask the athlete if he/she could flex or extend the knee?

Did you perform a Lachman test for possible anterior cruciate injury?

3A. Did you remove the individual from the court with a two-person assistive carry?

During the off-the-court evaluation, did you:
  - repeat the history
  - further observe and palpate the injury
  - have the athlete flex and extend the knee, looking for limitations in range of motion and noting when pain occurred
  - repeat the Lachman test
  - perform valgus stress test for medial collateral ligament, menisci test, and other test that might indicate injury to associated structures

3B. Did you suspect an injury to the anterior cruciate ligament? Did you suspect other medial structures may be damaged because of the mechanism of injury and their close anatomical association with the anterior cruciate? Did the management plan include:
  - ice, compression, and elevation
  - fitting the individual for crutches
  - immobilizing the limb in an appropriate brace
  - physician referral

4 **Osteochondritis Dissecans**

During the special test, did you:
- test bilaterally
- have the individual flex and extend the knee noting pain and limitations in range of motion
- look for locking during range of motion
- perform resistive range of motion testing that included extension and external rotation as well as extension and internal rotation

4A. Because of the age of this sport participant and the findings discovered during the evaluation, did you suspect this injury to be osteochondritis dissecans?

Did your management plan include physician referral for further evaluation and radiographs

 Patellofemoral Stress Syndrome

During the history, did you ask:
- what, where, when, and how questions
- about previous injury, medications, treatment
- about type of pain
- functional abilities
- if rest helps
- about changes in training and running surface
- footwear

During observation, did you observe bilaterally for:
- swelling, deformity, discoloration, other signs of trauma
- pes planus, pes cavus, foot pronation, foot supination
- genu varus, genu valgus, tibial torsion, patella alta
- leg length discrepancies
- gait pattern
- footwear

5A. During palpation, did you palpate bilaterally for:
- swelling, point tenderness, deformity, crepitation, temperature, other signs of trauma
- patello femoral joint pain

During the special tests, did you:
- do bilateral comparison
- assess strength of vastus medialis oblique
- passively extend and flex the knee while your hand was on the patella, noting any crepitation
- resistive knee extension, noting pain
- passively extend and flex the knee, observing for laterally patellar deviation
- do the patella compression test or Waldron's test
- have the individual squat or perform a duck walk

Did you suspect this individual has patello femoral syndrome?

Did you determine that the following conditions may have contributed to her condition?
- changes in training and surface
- postural abnormalities
- laterally patella deviation
- strength of vastus medialis oblique
(Refer to pages 291–293 in the text.)

V. Situations

l. Acute Prepatella Bursitis - Did you determine that the wrestler could have acute prepatella bursitis and that this is an extraarticular injury? Did your management plan include:
- ice, compression, elevation
- decrease in activity
- NSAIDS
- referral to physician to rule out infectious bursitis if the skin has been broken over the injured area
(Refer to pages 282–283 in the text)

2. Iliotibial Band Syndrome - Did you suspect the runner's condition to be iliotibial band syndrome? Did you include these factors that can predispose someone to iliotibial band syndrome?
- changes in training, surface, footwear
- excessive Q-angle
- gender
- postural abnormalities
- running on the same side of the road
- hill running or stair running
(Refer to Field Strategy 8-5 on pages 297–299 for management protocol)

3. Medial Menisci Injury - Did you perform McMurry's test and the Apley compression test to determine if the softball player had a menisci injury? During your rational for completing the tests, did you explain how both tests were attempting to recreate the mechanism of injury in pinching the menisci between the tibia and femur? A positive test would produce pain and clicking.
(Refer to pages 289–291 in text.)

4. Dislocated Patella - In the management plan, did you include the following?
- ice, compression, and elevation
- immobilization in the position you found the athlete in
- immediate physician referral to reduce the dislocation

Did you determine that the following structures could also be injured because of this injury?
- medial muscular attachments
- retinaculum attachments
- patellar fracture or lateral femoral condyle

5. Osgood-Schlatter Disease - In determining the difference between Osgood-Schlatter disease and patella tendinitis, did you:
- palpate the tibial tuberosity and patella tendon for pain to determine which structure was injured.
(Refer to pages 296–297 for treatment protocols)

6. Nonweight-Bearing Exercises - **Refer to page 314 in the text** - Did the you have the individual perform the following nonweight-bearing exercises?
- quadriceps contractions
- straight leg raises in hip flexion, extension, abduction, and adduction
- short arc knee extensions

VI. Special Tests
Refer to pages 306–313 in the text

VII. Multiple Choice Answers

1. c	8. d	15. a
2. b	9. c	16. c
3. a	10. b	17. c
4. b	11. a	18. b
5. c	12. b	19. c
6. b	13. d	20. d
7. d	14. c	

Chapter 9 Thigh, Hip and Pelvis Injuries

After completing this chapter you should be able to:

- Locate the important bony and soft tissue structures of the thigh, hip, and pelvis

- Describe the motions of the hip and identify muscles that produce them

- Explain what forces produce loading patterns responsible for common injuries of the thigh, hip, and pelvis

- Recognize specific injuries of the thigh, hip, and pelvis

- Demonstrate an assessment of the hip region

- Identify protective padding and commercial products to assist in the prevention and management of injuries to the thigh, hip, and pelvis

- Demonstrate general rehabilitation exercises for the region

I. Anatomy Review

Materials Needed:
-SKELETON   -ANATOMICAL THIGH, HIP, AND PELVIS CHARTS   -NONPERMANENT MARKERS

Instructions: *Work with a partner to perform the following:*
- *identify the following anatomical structures on the skeleton or anatomical charts.*
- *palpate and draw the anatomical structures on your partner using the nonpermanent markers.*

─── Structures of the Thigh, Hip, and Pelvis ───

-femur	-zona orbicularis
-femoral neck	-iliopsoas bursa
-acetabulum	-deep trochanteric bursa
-ilium	-iliofemoral ligament
-ischium	-pubofemoral ligament
-pelvis	-ischofemoral ligament
-iliac crests	-rectus femoris
-anterior superior iliac spine (ASIS)	-iliopsoas
-posterior superior iliac spine (PSIS)	-sartorius
-pubis symphysis	-pectineus

-tensor fascia latae
-gluteus maximus, medius, and minimus
-gracilis
-adductor magnus, longus, and brevis
-semitendinosus
-semimembranosus

-biceps femoris
-lateral rotators
-lumbar plexus, femoral nerve, and obturator nerve
-sacral plexus, sciatic nerve
-femoral artery

II. Key Terms

Instructions: *Define the following terms.*

-Lumbar plexus
-Sacral plexus
-Forward and backward pelvic tilt
-Osteitis pubis
-Myositis ossificans
-Hip pointer

-Snapping hip syndrome
-Legg-Calvé-Perthes disease
-Osteochondrosis
-Thromoboplebitis
-Phlebothrombosis
-Pulmonary embolism

III. Kinematics of the Thigh, Hip, and Pelvis

Instructions: *Work with a partner to perform the following. Have your partner perform the following movements while you name the muscles that are performing the movements along with the normal range of motion for each movement.*

	Muscle	**Range of Motion**
-knee extension		
-knee flexion		
-hip extension		
-hip flexion		
-lateral rotation at the hip		
-medial rotation at the hip		
-abduction at the hip		
-adduction at the hip		

After you have determined range of motion of the hip through subjective means, measure both hip flexion and abduction using a goniometer.

IV. Simulations

Instructions: *Perform the following simulated experiences.*

A rugby player is down on the field after receiving a severe blow to the anterior right thigh. The thigh is externally rotated and severely angulated. Swelling is present, and the athlete is in severe pain. Demonstrate immediate action for this injury.

1A. The distal pulse is strong and regular. Skin color and temperature are normal. Have you treated the player for shock? What is the next step in the treatment of this injury?

Two weeks ago a football player received a severe blow to his right anterior thigh. He still complains of discomfort, lack of flexibility, and lack of full muscular contractions. Perform palpation.

2A. You find a hard mass over the injured area. What injury should you suspect? What treatment would you recommend? How would you prevent this injury from recurring in the future?

A 47-year-old woman is complaining of pain while running. Pain is localized on the posterolateral aspect of her hip near the greater trochanter and is occasionally accompanied by a snapping sensation. Perform a history and observation.

3A. The woman has been running more hilly surfaces lately and on the same side of a downward sloped road. She has a leg length discrepancy of one-half inch and an increased Q-angle on the affected leg. What structures could be involved? Please demonstrate special testing procedures.

3B. You find the runner has limited hamstring flexibility, lack of strength in hip abduction, and a positive Ober's test. What condition should be suspected? What treatment do you recommend?

4 A breastroker is complaining of sharp pain in the groin area. The swimmer reports sustaining an acute injury during slide board exercises. Explain and demonstrate special testing procedures.

4A. You find pain, stiffness, and weakness in hip adduction and flexion. Straight-ahead and side-to-side movements are extremely difficult. Increased pain occurs during passive stretching with the hip extended, abducted, and externally rotated. What injury should be suspected? If this injury was not acute and the swimmer had no pain during range of motion and special testing, but still had pain, what other anatomical structures could be involved?

V. Situations

Instructions: *Work with a partner to cooperatively analyze and address the following situations.*

1. During takeoff, a high jumper experiences a painful snap on the anterior side of the right iliac crest. Pain is increased during palpation of the anterior superior iliac spine, during active hip flexion, and while placing the ankle of the involved leg on the contralateral knee. What injury should be suspected? What treatment do you recommend?

2. An aerobic dancer is complaining of pain over the anterior groin that increases after weight-bearing activity but decreases with rest. The dancer does not recall a specific injury. Deep palpation in the inguinal area produces discomfort. What special testing procedures does this injury warrant? What injury should be suspected?

3. A soccer player received a direct blow to the left anterolateral thigh. Immediate pain, loss of function, and mild swelling are evident. Explain and demonstrate how swelling should be controlled.

4. A volleyball player was digging a ball and fell directly onto her anterior hip. Describe observation procedures and how you would differentiate between bone and muscular injury. Will the athlete need protective equipment to return to activity? If yes, what type will be needed?

5. A middle-distance runner is complaining of tightness and a pulling sensation just distal to the ischial tuberosity. It is uncomfortable when running on level ground, but painful and tight when running up hills. What muscle group may be injured? What special tests can be used to determine the severity of injury? What immediate treatment do you recommend? Explain and demonstrate flexibility exercises for the hamstrings.

V. Situations (Con't)

6. A softball player was struck on the medial side of the distal thigh with a line drive. Ice, compression, and elevation significantly reduced the initial swelling and discoloration. Several days later, the player is complaining of an aching, burning pain and superficial tenderness over the area. What can account for this delayed burning pain? What vascular structures may be damaged? What further treatment is necessary?

VI. Special Tests

Instructions: *Work with a partner to perform the following special tests, explaining the rationale for each test.*

- Gapping test
- Faber' or Patrick's test
- Thomas' test
- Lasègue's test (straight leg raising test)
- Leg length measurement

- Sign of the buttock test
- Ober' test
- Kendall's test
- Hamstring contracture test

VII. Multiple Choice Questions

Instructions: Choose the best answer for each question.

___1. The acetabular labrum deepens the hip socket and _____ to the joint.
    a. enhances movement   c. adds stability
    b. limits movement   d. decreases stability

___2. The zona arbicularis forms the _____ and contributes to _____.
    a. joint capsular fibers of the hip, joint stability
    b. joint capsular fibers of the hip, increased hip motion
    c. acetabular labrum, joint stability
    d. joint ligament, increased hip motion

___3. The Y-ligament of Bigelow strengthens the joint capsule_____.
    a. posteriorly   c. laterally
    b. anteriorly   d. in all planes of movement

___4. The peroneal and tibial nerves are branches of the ___ which is part of the _____.
    a. axillary nerve, brachial plexus   c. sciatic nerve, lumbar plexus
    b. long thoracic nerve, thoracic plexus.   d. sciatic nerve, sacral plexus

___5. Lack of circulation in the hamstring muscles would indicate an injury to the___.
    a. peroneal artery   c. axillary artery
    b. tibial artery   d. femoral artery

___6. The lateral rotator stretch aids in the stretching of the _____.
    a. hip flexor muscles   c. adductor muscles
    b. iliotibial band   d. hip extensor muscles

___7.   The most common site for a quadriceps contusion is the _____.
         a. anterolateral thigh   c. superior thigh near the groin
         b. anteromedial thigh   d. distal thigh near the patella

___8.   When applying ice to a quadriceps contusion or a hip pointer, the knee should be
         placed in ___.
         a. maximal extension   c. neutral position
         b. maximal flexion   d. a knee splint

___9.   An athlete received a blow to the anterior thigh 1 week ago. Upon reevaluation
         of the injury, your examination reveals a warm, firm, swollen thigh nearly 2 to
         4 cm larger than the unaffected thigh. Active quadriceps contractions and straight
         leg raises are limited. What injury do you suspect?
         a. myositis ossificans   c. fractured femur
         b. active hematoma   d. severe quadriceps strain

___10.   A runner reports to you with pain over the lateral hip that intensifies after
         exercise. Pain increases in intensity upon resistive hip abduction and during
         flexion and extension of the hip during weight bearing. What injury do you
         suspect?
         a. iliopsoas strain   c. sprain of the Y-ligament
         b. iliopsoas bursitis   d. greater trochanteric bursitis

___11.   Spasms in the _____ can compress the sciatic nerve leading to sciatic-
         like pain and symptoms.
         a. sartorius muscle   c. piriformis muscle
         b. iliopsoas muscle   d. rectus femoris muscle

___12.   The rectus femoris is often injured during _____.
         a. explosive knee flexion and hip extension movements
         b. explosive knee extension and hip flexion movements
         c. explosive hip flexion movements
         d. explosive hip abduction movements

___13.   Muscle atrophy of the _____ during chronic hamstring strains can lead to
         anterolateral knee instability.
         a. biceps femoris   c. semitendinosus
         b. semimembranosus   d. rectus femoris

___14.   Groin pain may be referred from all but which of the following?
         a. bladder   c. spleen
         b. testicle   d. sacroiliac joint

___15.   Legg-Calvé-Perthes disease is considered to be an osteochondrosis condition of
         the _____ and is often found in young children.
         a. iliac crest   c. greater trochanter
         b. femoral head   d. ischial tuberosity

___16.   Osteitis pubis is a stress fracture of the _____ caused by repeated overload
         of the _____.
         a. pubic symphysis, abductor muscle   c. femoral head, rectus femoris
         b. pubic symphysis, adductor muscle   d. ischial tuberosity, biceps femoris

_17. To determine a fracture to the pelvis you would _____.
   a. apply compression anteriorly and posteriorly to the ilium and ASIS
   b. apply compression to the sides of the ilium and ASIS
   c. send a longitudinal force through the ischium
   d. have the athlete jump up and down from a sitting position

_18. After sustaining a fracture to the femur an athlete's foot turns pale and cold. What do you suspect is occurring to this athlete?
   a. vascular deficits   c. neurological deficits
   b. shock   d. avascular necrosis

_19. To test for flexion contracture of the hip, _____ test can be used.
   a. Thompson's   c. Kendall's
   b. Thomas'   d. Lasègue's

_20. Pain that does not increase with dorsiflexion of the foot or neck flexion during a straight leg raise usually indicates _____.
   a. stretching of the dura mater of the spinal cord and nerve injury
   b. hamstring tightness with no associated nerve injury
   c. hamstring tightness with associated sciatic injury
   d. hip extensor tightness

VIII. Additional Activities

l. **Visit a physical therapy clinic and observe hip evaluations and rehabilitation exercises.**

2. **Develop a stretching and preventative exercise program for hip injuries.**

3. **Visit an athletic trainer that works with football and have them demonstrate how hip and thigh pads are used for the prevention of injuries.**

I. Anatomy

Refer to Table 9-1 on page 324 in the text

II. Key Terms

Anterior pelvic tilt — — — Anterior sagittal plane tilt of the ASIS with respect to the pubic symphysis

Posterior pelvic tilt — — — Posterior sagittal plane tilt of the ASIS with respect to the pubic symphysis

Lumbar plexus — — — — — Interconnected roots of the first four lumbar spinal nerves

Sacral plexus — — — — — Interconnected roots of the L_4-S_4 spinal nerves

Hip pointer — — — — — — Contusion caused by direct compression to an unprotected iliac crest that crushes soft tissue and sometimes the bone itself

Myositis ossificans — — — Ectopic ossification resulting in bone disposition within muscle tissue

Snapping hip syndrome — — A snapping sensation either heard or felt during motion of the hip

Osteitis pubis — — — — — Stress fracture of the pubic symphysis caused by repeated overload of the adductor muscles or repetitive stress activities

Osteochondrosis — — — — Any condition characterized by degeneration or aseptic necrosis of the articular cartilage due to limited blood supply

Legg-Calvé-Perthes disease - Avascular necrosis of the proximal femoral epiphysis seen especially in young males ages 3 to 8

Hypervolemic shock — — Shock caused by excessive loss of whole blood or plasma

Thrombophlebitis — — — Acute inflammation of a vein

Phlebothrombosis — — — Thrombosis, or clotting, in a vein without overt inflammatory signs or symptoms

Pulmonary embolism — — Occurs when a blood clot travels through the circulatory system to lodge in a blood vessel of the lungs

III. Kinematics of the Thigh, Hip and Pelvis

Movement	Muscles	Normal ROM
Knee extension	Rectus femoris	0–15°
Knee flexion	Semitendinosus	0–125°
	Semimembranosus	
	Biceps femoris	
Hip extension	Gluteus maximus	10–15°
	Semitendinosus	
	Semimembranosus	
	Biceps femoris	
Hip flexion	Rectus femoris	110–120°
	Pectineus	
	Iliopsoas	
Lateral hip rotation	Sartorius	40–60°
	Gluteus maximus	
Medial hip rotation	Tensor fascia latae	30–40°
	Gluteus minimus	
Hip abduction	Gluteus medius	30–50°
	Sartorius	
Hip adduction	Gracilis	30°
	Adductor magnus	
	Adductor longus	
	Adductor brevis	

Refer to Table 9-1 on page 324 in the text; Table 9-2 on page 328 in the text, and to page 347 in the text.

IV. Simulations

 Fractured Femur

(Refer to Table 9-4 on page 343 in the text)

Did you check the neurovascular function of the leg by checking for:
- a distal pulse
- skin color and other signs of shock
- for sensory changes through lower extremity dermatome function

1 Fractured Femur (Con't)

1A. Did you initiate the emergency medical plan by calling EMS, keep the player comfortable and in a stable position, and treat for shock? If bleeding is present, did you cover the area with a dry sterile dressing? Did you take vital signs and monitor the player's condition until the ambulance arrived?

2 Myositis Ossificans

Did you palpate bilaterally for:
- point tenderness, swelling, muscle spasms and deformity
- hardness or a firm mass
- an increase in skin temperature

2A. Did you suspect myositis ossificans? Did the management plan include:
- ICE
- crutches
- rest
- referral to a physician for follow-up treatment, radiographs, and prescribed NSAIDS

To prevent this condition from recuring, did you determine that the football player should:
- not return to activity before the contusion is healed
- wear protective padding

3 Snapping Hip Syndrome

Did you include questions about:
- present medications and treatment
- past injuries and treatment
- type of pain
- conditioning program
- type of surface
- type of shoes
- type of activities that increase and decrease pain
(Refer to Field Strategy 9-3 on page 345 in the text)

Did you observe bilaterally for:
- deformity, swelling, discoloration, muscle spasms, or other signs of trauma
- shoe wear
- lower extremity posture including pes cavus and planus, genu valgus and varus, tibial torsion, leg length discrepancy, and foot pronation or supination
- Q-angle
- walking and running gait pattern

(Refer to Field Strategy 9-4 on page 346 in the text)

3A. Did you determine that the greater trochanteric bursa and iliotibial band could be involved in this injury?

Did your special tests include:
- active, passive, and resistive range of motion of the hip and knee
- hamstring flexibility
- Ober's test

3B. Did you suspect snapping hip syndrome? Did the management plan include ice, modification of activity, NSAIDS, and flexibility exercises?

4   **Groin Strain**

(Refer to Table 9-4 on page 343 in the text)

Did your special tests include:
- passive, active, and resistive range of motion at the hip
- weight-bearing activity (running and side sliding)

4A. Did you suspect a groin strain? If the swimmer had not reported an acute injury, did you suspect injury to the following structures?
- bowel
- bladder
- testicle
- kidney
- abdomen

V. Situations

l. Avulsion Fracture of the Anterior Superior Iliac Spine - (Refer to Table 9-4 on page 343 in the text) - Did you suspect an avulsion fracture of the anterior superior iliac spine? Did your immediate treatment plan include ice, rest, and use of crutches?

2. Stress Fracture of the Pubis, Femoral Neck, or Proximal Third of Femur - (Refer to table 9-4 on page 343 in the text) - During special testing, did you note increased pain on hip rotation and an inability to stand on the involved leg? Did you suspect a stress fracture to either the pubis, femoral neck, or proximal third of the femur?

3. Anterior Thigh Contusion - To control swelling, reduce intramuscular bleeding and spasm, did you apply ice with the thigh in 120 degrees of flexion?

4. Hip Pointer - Did you observe bilaterally for swelling, deformity, discoloration, or loss of function? To determine between muscle and bone injury did you:
  - palpate the iliac crest and surrounding musculature
  - perform passive, active, and resistive range of motion exercises
  - perform weight-bearing exercises

Did you suspect a contusion of the iliac crest or a hip pointer?
Did you apply a donut type of padding to prevent further aggravation?

5. Hamstring Strain - (Refer to Table 9-3 on page 336 in the text) - Did you determine that the hamstring muscle group may be involved because of its attachment to the ischial tuberosity? Did your special testing include:
  - passive, active, and resistive range of motion
  - functional testing (walking, jumping, running)

Did you determine that the more resistance the individual could handle during resistive stress testing, the more mild the injury? Did your management plan include ice, compression, elevation, and mild stretching? Did you demonstrate static stretching exercises for the hamstrings?

6. Vascular Disorder - Did you determine that the softball player could be experiencing a vascular disorder to the arteries and veins that course through the injured area, particularly the femoral artery and vein? Did further treatment include an immediate referral to a physician?

VI. Special Testing

Refer to pages 346–356 in the text

VII. Multiple Choice Answers

1. c	8. b	15. b
2. a	9. a	16. b
3. b	10. d	17. b
4. d	11. c	18. a
5. d	12. b	19. b
6. b	13. a	20. b
7. a	14. c	

Chapter 10 Shoulder Injuries

After completing this chapter you should be able to:

- Locate important bony and soft tissue structures of the shoulder

- Describe the major motions at the shoulder and identify muscles that produce them

- Explain the forces that produce the loading patterns responsible for common injuries in the shoulder

- Recognize and describe specific injuries in the shoulder region

- Describe management protocol for specific injuries in the shoulder region

- Demonstrate a thorough assessment of the shoulder

- Demonstrate proper fitting of football shoulder pads

- Identify protective equipment or pads used to protect the shoulder region from injury

- Demonstrate general rehabilitation exercises for the shoulder complex

I. Anatomy Review

Materials Needed:
-Skeleton   -Anatomical shoulder charts   -Nonpermanent markers

Instructions: *Work with a partner to perform the following:*
- identify the following anatomical structures on the skeleton or anatomical charts.
- palpate and draw the anatomical structures on your partner using the nonpermanent marker.

Structures of the Shoulder

-humerus   -coracoclavicular joint
-scapula   -glenohumeral joint
-clavicle   -scapulothoracic joint
-sternum   -glenoid fossa
-sternoclavicular joint   -glenoid labrum
-acromioclavicular joint   -subcoracoid bursa

-subscapularis bursa
-subacromial bursa
-anterior deltoid
-middle deltoid
-posterior deltoid
-pectoralis major
-subscapularis
-supraspinatus
-infraspinatus
-teres minor
-teres major
-latissimus dorsi

-coracobrachialis
-long head biceps brachii
-short head biceps brachii
-triceps brachii
-axillary nerve
-musculocutaneous nerve
-dorsal scapular nerve
-subscapular nerve
-suprascapular nerve
-pectoral nerve
-subclavian artery
-axillary artery

II. Key Terms

Instructions: *Define the following terms.*

-Brachial plexus
-Glenoid labrum
-Rotator cuff
-Little league shoulder
-Bankart lesion

-Dead arm syndrome
-Impingement syndrome
-Thoracic outlet syndrome
-Scapulohumeral rhythm

III. Kinematics of the Shoulder

Instructions: *Work with a partner to perform the following. Have your partner perform the following movements while you name the muscles that are performing the movements along with the normal range of motion for each movement.*

	Muscle	**Normal ROM**
-flexion of the arm	_____	_____
-extension of the arm	_____	_____
-abduction	_____	_____
-adduction	_____	_____
-horizontal abduction or horizontal extension	_____	_____
-horizontal adduction or horizontal flexion	_____	_____
-internal or medial rotation	_____	_____
-external or lateral rotation	_____	_____
-scapulohumeral rhythm	_____	_____

After range of motion has been subjectively measured, use a goniometer to measure both shoulder flexion and abduction.

IV. Simulations

Instructions: *Perform the following simulated experiences.*

A young gymnast lost her balance on a dismount and fell onto the point of the right shoulder. Observation reveals the shoulder sagging downward and forward. There is a visible lump in the midclavicular region. Perform palpation and special testing.

1A. Palpation reveals muscle spasms, pain over the midclavicular area, and a positive piano key sign. Explain and demonstrate the immediate treatment protocol for this injury.

A basketball player received a blow to his left superior shoulder. The player is complaining of pain over the acromioclavicular joint. Perform observation and palpation.

2A. Observation reveals an overriding clavicle on the acromion of the affected shoulder. There is minor swelling over the joint line but no discoloration. Palpation reveals a mobile clavicle as you press down on it and it pops back up. There are no other signs of trauma. What injury should be suspected? Explain and demonstrate the immediate treatment protocol for this injury.

A swimmer reports to the training room complaining of anterior shoulder pain. Perform a history.

3A. You determine that this is a chronic injury. The swimmer reports feeling a subluxation during the power phase of both the crawl and butterfly stroke. Continue the evaluation.

3B. Palpation reveals tenderness along the anterior and the posterior glenohumeral joint. During active shoulder abduction and external rotation, a clicking feeling and discomfort are felt. During anterior and posterior stress to the glenohumeral joint, you find considerable laxity as compared to the uninjured shoulder. What anatomical structures could be involved? What injury should you suspect?

A baseball pitcher reports to you with chronic pain over his right anterior shoulder. Perform observation.

4A. Observation reveals minor swelling, no discoloration, or deformity. However, you do find the right shoulder to be slightly lower than the left when viewed from the posterior. During palpation, point tenderness is elicited over the head of the humerus. Perform range of motion and special testing for this injury.

V. Situations

Instructions: *Work with a partner to cooperatively analyze and address the following situations.*

1. A little league pitcher is complaining of shoulder pain. He does not recall having an acute injury; however, he is now bothered with pain and discomfort during his pitching activity. Palpation elicits pain in the axilla region. There is minor discomfort with anterior shoulder palpation. What injury should be suspected? Why? What treatment do you recommend?

2. A baseball player is complaining that his right shoulder feels "dead" in the cocking phase of the throwing motion. Pain increases during acceleration. Muscular endurance and strength are not at the level earlier in the season. Palpation during abduction and external rotation reveals a clicking sensation. What structures may be involved in this injury? What treatment do you recommend?

3. A quarterback received a blow to his throwing arm after releasing the ball during a pass. The shoulder was forced into excessive abduction, external rotation, and extension. During palpation, you find the head of the humerus to be sitting anterior of the glenoid fossa. What injury should be suspected? Would you further palpate for neurological functioning? If yes, demonstrate this procedure. What treatment do you recommend?

4. A volleyball player reports severe pain during overhand hitting drills that is getting progressively worse. The individual is unable to actively abduct the arm between 70 and 120 degrees without pain. What structures do you suspect to be involved? Explain and demonstrate special tests. How would you differentiate between bursitis and tendinitis?

5. A freestyle sprint swimmer reports anterior shoulder pain that increases concomitantly with more intense workouts. There is a clicking feeling when moving through the pull phase of the freestyle stroke. During observation and palpation, you find diffuse swelling and point tenderness under the acromion and along the insertion of the supraspinatus. Movement is restricted during shoulder abduction. Explain and demonstrate special testing for this injury. What treatment do you recommend?

6. A tennis player complains of pain in his anterior upper arm. The athlete does not recall an injury. Pain and point tenderness are felt over the bicipital groove during internal and external rotation of the shoulder. How would you passively stretch the structure that passes through the bicipital groove? What injury should be suspected? What treatment do you recommend?

VI. Special Tests

Instructions: *Work with a partner to explain and demonstrate the rationale for the following shoulder tests:*

- Wall push-up
- Acromioclavicular distraction and compression test
- Apprehension test
- Drop arm test
- Centinela supraspinatus muscle test

- Anterior impingement test
- Transverse ligament test
- Yergason's test
- Speed's test
- Thoracic outlet compression syndrome test

VII. Multiple Choice Questions

Instructions: Choose the best answer for each question.

___1. The coracoclavicular joint is a _____formed by the binding together of the coracoid process of the scapula and the inferior surface of the clavicle by the coracoclavicular ligament.
a. diathrotic joint   c. synovial joint
b. syndesmosis   d. hinge joint

___2. The _____ hold the head of the humerus in the glenoid fossa and produce humeral rotation.
a. deltoid muscle   c. acromioclavicular ligament
b. glenoid labrum   d. SITS muscles

___3. The _____ bursa may become irritated when repeatedly compressed during the overhand arm action.
a. subacromial   c. subcoracoid
b. subscapularis   d. subdeltoid

___4. Motion at the glenohumeral joint takes place in the _____.
   a. sagittal plane   c. frontal plane
   b. transverse plane   d. all three planes

___5. Scapulohumeral movement contributes to approximately _____ of the total rotational movement of the humerus.
   a. 50%   c. 25%
   b. 33%   d. 10%

___6. Maximum shearing force of the glenohumeral joint has been found when the arm is _____ to approximately _____.
   a. rotated, 60 degrees   c. elevated, 60 degrees
   b. rotated, 90 degrees   d. elevated, 90 degrees

___7. To strengthen the supraspinatus muscle, light resistance exercises can be done _____.
   a. in the first 30 degrees of abduction
   b. in the first 30 degrees of adduction
   c. through full abduction/rotation movement
   d. in all planes of movement

___8. After receiving a blow to the sternum area, an athlete is having difficulty in swallowing, diminished pulse, and hoarseness. What injury may have occurred?
   a. glenohumeral joint dislocation
   b. anterior displacement of the clavicle
   c. posterior displacement of the clavicle
   d. fracture of the sternum

___9. With an acromioclavicular separation, the _____ is elevated.
   a. distal clavicle   c. scapula
   b. proximal clavicle   d. deltoid muscle

___10. During a glenohumeral dislocation, it is imperative to assess both the _____ and _____ to determine neurovascular functioning.
   a. subclavian artery and axillary nerve   c. axillary artery and axillary nerve
   b. axillary artery and suprascapular nerve d. subclavian artery and radial nerve

___11. Dead arm syndrome is associated with _____.
   a. shoulder impingement   c. acromioclavicular separation
   b. recurrent anterior shoulder dislocations d. frozen shoulder syndrome

___12. Pain during glenohumeral abduction of the arm between 70 and 120 degrees is termed _____ and is associated with _____.
   a. painful arc, glenohumeral dislocations
   b. painful arc, impingement syndrome
   c. MDI, recurrent shoulder subluxation
   d. MDI, torn supraspinatus muscle

___13. Pain and tenderness over the bicipital groove when the shoulder is internally and externally rotated may be indicative of _____.
   a. thoracic outlet syndrome   c. biceps tendon rupture
   b. rotator cuff tendinitis   d. bicipital tendinitis

___14. Numbness in the side of the neck that extends across the shoulder down the medial arm to the ulnar aspect of the hand, along with weakness in grasp and atrophy in hand muscles, may lead one to suspect _____.
   a. rotator cuff tear
   b. cervical plexus injury
   c. thoracic outlet compression syndrome
   d. posterior glenohumeral dislocation

___15. An athlete approaches you with their head turned to the right side and supporting their right arm with their left arm. What type of injury do you suspect?
   a. scapular fracture   c. brachial plexus injury
   b. clavicular fracture   d. glenohumeral dislocation

___16. The mechanism of injury for little league shoulder is most often _____.
   a. direct trauma   c. compression force
   b. repetitive rotational stress d. repetitive compressive stress

___17. Intra-articular swelling would prevent the athlete from _____.
   a. fully adducting the arm   c. abducting the arm
   b. externally rotating the arm d. extending the arm

___18. Crepitus about the shoulder could indicate all but which of the following?
   a. inflamed subacromial bursa   c. irregular articular surface
   b. bicipital tenosynovitis   d. deltoid myositis ossificans

___19. The _____ is associated with serratus anterior weakness or winged scapula.
   a. long thoracic nerve   c. subthoracic nerve
   b. rhomboid muscle   d. pectoralis nerve

___20. The drop arm test is used to determine _____.
   a. glenohumeral dislocation
   b. bicipital tendinitis
   c. integrity of the supraspinatus muscle
   d. integrity of the subscapularis tendon

VIII. Additional Activities

l. Visit a nearby college and ask the athletic trainer for baseball to demonstrate various shoulder evaluation techniques.

2. Develop a rehabilitation program for a rotator cuff injury to an athlete who throws overhand.

3. Demonstrate how you would immobilize and treat an anterior shoulder dislocation and a second degree acromioclavicular sprain.

4. Visit a nearby orthopedic or medical facility and ask if they would demonstrate the various supportive devices used for shoulder injuries.

5. Analyze the overhand throwing motion and determine the types of injury that may occur during each phase.

Student's Key

I. Anatomy Review

Refer to Table 10-1 on page 368 in the text.

II. Key Terms

Brachial plexus — — — — A complex web of spinal nerves (C_5-T_1) that innervate the upper extremity

Glenoid labrum — — — — Soft tissue lip around the periphery of the glenoid fossa that adds stability to the glenohumeral joint

Rotator cuff — — — — — — The SITS muscles (supraspinatus, infraspinatus, teres minor, and subscapularis) hold the head of the humerus in the glenoid fossa and produce humeral rotation

Little league shoulder — — Fracture of the proximal humeral growth plate in adolescents caused by repetitive rotational stresses during the act of pitching

Bankart lesion — — — — — Avulsion or damage to the anterior lip of the glenoid as the humerus slides forward in an anterior dislocation

Dead arm syndrome — — — Common sensation felt with a recurrent anterior shoulder dislocation

Impingement syndrome — Chronic condition caused by repetitive overhead activity that damages the glenoid labrum, long head of the biceps brachii, and subacromial bursa

Thoracic outlet syndrome — Condition whereby nerves and/or vessels become compressed in the root of the neck or axilla, leading to numbness in the arm

Scapulohumeral rhythm — Coordinated rotational movement of the scapula that accompanies abduction and adduction of the humerus

III. Kinematics

Refer to Table 10-1 on page 368 in the text; Table 10-2 on page 374 in the text; and page 402 in text.

Movement	Muscles	Normal ROM
Flexion of the arm	Anterior deltoid	160–180°
	Pectoralis major	
Extension of the arm	Posterior deltoid	50–60°
	Latissimus dorsi	
Abduction	Middle deltoid	170–180°
	Supraspinatus	
Adduction	Biceps brachii	50–70°
	Triceps brachii	
	Latissimus dorsi	
Horizontal abduction/extension	Posterior deltoid	130°
	Infraspinatus	
	Middle deltoid	
Horizontal adduction/flexion	Anterior deltoid	130°
	Pectoralis major	
Internal/medial rotation	Teres major	60–100°
	Subscapularis	
External/lateral rotation	Teres minor	80–90°
	Infraspinatus	
Scapulohumeral rhythm	Triceps	
	Rhomboids	
	Serratus anterior	
	Levator scapula	

IV. Simulations

 Fractured Clavicle

During palpation, did you palpate the following structures for point tenderness, swelling, deformity, crepitation, muscle spasms, sensation, and other signs of trauma?
- deltoid
- acromion process
- scapula
- trapezius
- clavicle
- pectoralis muscles
- sternum
- coracoid process

1   Fractured Clavicle (Con't)

Did you do bilateral comparisons?

During special testing, did you:
- perform range of motion exercises
- push down on the clavicle to determine stability

1A. Did you determine that the gymnast may have a fractured clavicle? Immediate treatment should include immobilization through the use of a sling and swathe, ice, and physician referral.

2   Acromioclavicular Sprain

Refer to Field Strategy 10-4 on page 382 in the text

During observation, did you bilaterally observe for swelling, deformity, discoloration, and other signs of trauma.

During palpation, did you palpate the following structures for point tenderness, swelling, deformity, crepitation, muscles spasms, and other signs of trauma?
- deltoid
- scapula
- clavicle
- acromion process
- coracoid process
- sternum
- pectoralis muscles
- trapezius
- joint line

2A. Did you determine that the basketball player could have an injury to the acromioclavicular ligament? Immediate treatment should include ice, compression, and elevation. During the history, did you determine if the injury was chronic or acute?

Refer to Field Strategy 10-8 on page 400 in the text and to page 385 in the text.

Did you ask:
- where, when, and how questions
- about training regimen (time, distance, progression)
- about type of swimming stroke
- about pain (type, frequency, duration, radiating, referred, intensity)
- about previous injuries and treatment rendered
- if the athlete is taking any medications

3A. During palpation, did you palpate the following structures for point tenderness, swelling, deformity, crepitation, sensation, and other signs of trauma bilaterally?
- clavicle
- scapula
- humerus
- acromion process
- coracoid process
- subacromial space
- glenohumeral joint
- deltoid
- rotator cuff muscles
- pectoralis muscles
- trapezius
- sensory at axillary nerve

During the special tests, did you perform the following bilaterally?
- passive, active, and resistive range of motion testing
- anterior and posterior stress testing to the glenohumeral joint
- apprehension test

Did you notice any limits in range of motion, pain, or weakness?

3B. Since the injury was chronic, it could be a recurrent dislocation or subluxation of the glenohumeral joint. Did you determine that the humerus, glenoid fossa, glenoid labrum, rotator cuff muscles, and anterior glenohumeral ligaments could be involved?

Did you observe the following structures for swelling, deformity, discoloration, and other signs of trauma bilaterally? Was an upper body posture completed?
- clavicle
- scapula
- humerus
- acromion process
- acromioclavicular joint
- anterior and posterior soft tissue structures

4A. During the special tests, did you perform the following bilaterally?
- passive, active, and resistive range of motion
- drop arm test
- centinela supraspinatus muscle test

Did you notice any limitation in range of motion, pain, or weakness?

V. Situations

l. Little League Shoulder Injury - Because of no previous injury, pain upon throwing, pain upon palpation of the axillary region, and age of the athlete, did you determine that this injury could be Little league shoulder? Did your treatment protocol include immediate physician referral?

2. Recurrent Glenohumeral Subluxation or Glenoid Labrum Tear - Did you determine that the following anatomical structures could be injured?
- glenohumeral joint
- glenoid fossa
- glenoid labrum
- rotator cuff muscles
- anterior glenohumeral ligaments

Did the management of this injury include:
- ice
- physician referral
- stretching and strengthening program

3. Glenohumeral Dislocation - Did you determine that the quarterback may have a glenohumeral dislocation? As a result, you should check for a radial pulse and neurological function of the axillary nerve by checking sensation over the middle deltoid. Did the management plan include immobilization of the shoulder and arm, application of ice, and immediate referral to a physician?

4. Impingement Syndrome - Refer to pages 389 to 391 in the text - Did you determine that the following structures could be involved with this injury?
- rotator cuff muscles
- subacromial bursa
- subacromial space tissue
- biceps tendon

Did you perform the following special tests?
- passive, active, and resistive range of motion
- painful arc movement
- anterior impingement test

During range of motion, did you notice limits in movement, pain, and weakness?

5. Supraspinatus Strain - Refer to pages 388 to 389 and 408 and 411 in the text - Did you perform the following special tests?
- passive, active, and resistive range of motion
- drop arm test
- centinela supraspinatus muscle test

Did you suspect an injury to the supraspinatus? Did the treatment protocol include ice, rest, NSAIDS, modification of activity, and stretching and strengthening exercises?

6. Biceps Tendonitis - Refer to page 393 in the text - Did you passively stretch the biceps tendon by extending the shoulder with the elbow extended? This injury could be biceps tendonitis, and the treatment protocol should include ice, rest, NSAIDS, modification of activity, and stretching and strengthening exercises.

VI. Special Tests
Refer to pages 402–414 in text

VII. Multiple Choice Answers

l. b	8. c	15. b
2. d	9. a	16. b
3. a	10. c	17. a
4. d	11. b	18. d
5. b	12. b	19. a
6. c	13. d	20. c
7. a	14. c	

Chapter 11 — Upper Arm, Elbow and Forearm Injuries

After completing this chapter you should be able to:

- Locate the important bony and soft tissue structures in the upper arm, elbow, and forearm

- Describe the motions at the elbow and identify muscles that produce them

- Explain what forces produce loading patterns responsible for common injuries in the upper arm, elbow, and forearm

- Recognize and manage common injuries in the upper arm, elbow, and forearm.

- Demonstrate a thorough assessment of the elbow region

- Demonstrate common conditioning exercises for the elbow

I. Anatomy Review

Materials Needed:

SKELETON   ANATOMICAL SHOULDER CHARTS   NONPERMANENT MARKERS

Instructions: *Work with a partner to perform the following:*
- *identify the following anatomical structures on the skeleton or anatomical charts.*
- *palpate and draw the anatomical structures on your partner using the nonpermanent marker.*

─────────────── Anatomical Structures ───────────────

-humerus	-biceps brachii
-ulna	-brachioradialis
-radius	-brachialis
-olecranon	-pronator teres
-medial epicondyle	-pronator quadratus
-lateral epicondyle	-triceps brachii
-capitellum	-anconeus
-olecranon fossa	-supinator
-radial head	-olecranon bursa
-sulcus groove	-musculocutaneous nerve
-humeroulnar joint	-median nerve
-humeroradial joint	-ulnar nerve
-proximal radioulnar joint	-radial nerve

-brachial artery   -radial artery
-ulnar artery

II. Key Terms ────────────────────────────────
Instructions: *Define the following terms.*

Epicondylitis	Nightstick fracture	Pronator syndrome
Carrying angle	Ectopic bone	Wrist drop
Volkmann's contracture	Tackler's exostosis	Forearm splints
Monteggia's fracture	Periostitis	Cubital valgus
Galeazzi's fracture	Fibrositis	Cubital varus
Colles' fracture	Malaise	Resting position
Smith's fracture	Little leaguer's elbow	

III. Kinematics of the Upper Arm, Elbow, and Forearm ────────

Instructions: *Work with a partner to perform the following. Have your partner perform the following movements while you name the muscles that are performing the movements along with the normal range of motion for each movement.*
(Refer to pages 421-424 in text)

	Muscle	**Range of Motion**
- elbow flexion	_____	_____
- elbow extension	_____	_____
- forearm supination	_____	_____
- forearm pronation	_____	_____

After you have determined the range of motion of the elbow and forearm through subjective means, you should measure flexion of the elbow with the use of the goniometer

IV. Simulations ────────────────────────────────
Instructions: *Perform the following simulated experiences.*

1 **A tennis player is complaining of pain on the lateral side of the elbow that is exacerbated during the execution of ground strokes. Perform palpations by stating what anatomical structures could possibly be involved with this injury.**

IA. After palpating the lateral epicondyle and associated surrounding tissue and musculature, you found point tenderness over the proximal attachment of the wrist extensors, mild swelling, but no deformity. Continue with range of motion and special tests. How you will treat this injury?

A football player is complaining of pain on impact with his right forearm during blocking. History reveals an acute injury. Perform the observation and palpation procedures.

2A. After observing and palpating the area, you found no deformity or discoloration. There is, however, marked swelling and a hardend mass of soft tissue over the distal anterior arm. What injury might you suspect, and how would you treat this injury?

 A little league baseball player is complaining of pain on the medial elbow during pitching. Complete a history for this specific injury.

3A. You discovered that pain intensifies during the acceleration phase of throwing, although the throwing technique appears normal. Observation reveals minor swelling over the medial epicondyle. Please continue the evaluation with bilateral palpation and special tests. What nerve might be associated with this injury? What elbow injury do you suspect?

V. Situations

Instructions: *Work with a partner to cooperatively analyze and address the following situations.*

l. An athlete has sustained a supracondylar fracture of the left elbow region. What major complication may occur with this injury? How would you assess this condition?

2. A gymnast lost his hand position on a giant swing on the horizontal bar and fell to the floor on an outstretched arm. Immediate pain and deformity is evident along the distal forearm. How will you assess this condition to rule out injury to the neurovascular structures of the arm?

3. A wrestler has acute swelling about an inch in diameter on the proximal posterior ulna. His history reveals constant friction to the area. What condition do you suspect, what anatomical structures are involved, and how will you manage this condition?

4. A softball player, when sliding head first into second base, jammed an outstretched arm into the base. Observation reveals a noticeable posterior deformity of the elbow. The athlete is unwilling to move the elbow and is in extreme pain. Explain and demonstrate how to perform circulatory andneurological assessment of this injury. What immediate first-aid care would you render?

V. Situations (Con't)

5. After receiving a severe blow to the forearm, a lineman is having problems flexing his wrist and fingers. There is rapid swelling, discoloration and a diminished distal pulse. Passive stretching of the wrist flexors causes increased pain. What condition do you suspect and what anatomical structures are involved with this injury?

VI. Special Tests

Instructions: *Work with a partner to perform the following special tests and explain the rational for each test.*

- Valgus stress test
- Common extensor tendinitis test
- Tinel's sign
- Pinch grip test

- Varus stress test
- Medial epicondylitis test
- Elbow flexion test for ulnar neuritis

VII. Multiple Choice Questions

Instructions: Choose the best answer for each question.

___1. The hinge joint at the elbow is the:
a. humeroradial joint
b. humeroulnar joint
c. ulnaradial joint
d. trochlea-radial joint

___2. Forearm pronation and supination occur about a _____ joint at the elbow.
a. gliding
b. multiaxial
c. hinge
d. pivot

___3. The carrying angle ranges from _____ in adults and is generally greater in females.
a. 0 to 5 degrees
b. 5 to 10 degrees
c. 10 to 15 degrees
d. 15 to 20 degrees

___4. To test sensory function of the radial nerve, you would:
a. check sensation of the thumb
b. check sensation of the little finger
c. check strength of the thumb
d. check strength of the little finger

___5. The brachial artery can be palpated:
a. on the posterior surface of the elbow
b. on the anterior surface of the elbow
c. on the anterior surface of the wrist
d. on the posterior surface of the wrist

___6. The biceps brachii contributes most effectively to flexion when the forearm is _____ because it is slightly stretched.
a. extended
b. flexed
c. pronated
d. supinated

___7. The primary elbow flexor is the:
a. brachialis
b. brachioradialis
c. tricep long head
d. anconeus

___8. _____ are commonly used in racquet sports to reduce muscle tensile forces that can lead to medial or lateral epicondylitis.
a. neoprene sleeves
b. counterforce braces
c. compression wraps
d. elbow pads

___9.   Fractures and dislocations of the elbow usually occur because of:
         a. falling on an outstretched arm   c. repetitive stress
         b. direct blow   d. varus stress

___10. Contusion of the radial nerve during a blow to the elbow will exhibit signs of:
         a. transitory paralysis of the flexors of the forearm
         b. transitory paralysis of the extensors of the forearm
         c. sensory deficit of the middle finger
         d. sensory deficit of the ring and middle finger

___11. All of the following are used in the treatment of contusions except:
         a. ice, compression, and elevation   c. NSAIDS
         b. gentle range of motion without pain   d. aggressive stretching

___12. Acute anterior capsulitis of the elbow is often a result of:
         a. hyperextension injury   c. direct trauma
         b. chronic repetitive throwing   d. repetitive friction

___13. Dislocations of the elbow are second to:
         a. patella dislocations   c. glenohumeral dislocations
         b. proximal phalanx dislocations   d. distal phalanx dislocations

___14. The _____ is often ruptured during an elbow dislocation.
         a. anconeus muscle   c. radial collateral ligament
         b. fibrous cartilage   d. ulnar collateral ligament

___15. Most elbow dislocations occur in a _____ direction.
         a. anterior   c. varus
         b. posterior   d. valgus

___16. A positive valgus stress test at 15 to 20 degrees of elbow flexion often indicates:
         a. a tear to the radial collateral ligament   c. a tear to the biceps brachii
         b. a tear to the ulnar collateral ligament   d. a tear to the supinators

___17. Valgus stress forces frequently lead to:
         a. flexor-pronator muscle strain   c. radial collateral ligament injury
         b. extensor-supinator muscle strain   d. anterior capsulitits

___18. Little leaguer's elbow is a _____ injury.
         a. compression   c. tension stress
         b. shearing force   d. rotational

___19. Common extensor tendinitis is another term used for:
         a. medial epicondylitis   c. anterior capsulitis
         b. lateral epicondylitis   d. tricep synovitis

___20. During pronator syndrome, the _____ nerve is entrapped by the
         pronator teres, leading to pain on activities involving pronation.
         a. radial   c. brachial
         b. musculocutaneous   d. median

VIII. Additional Activities

1. Design a functional progressive throwing program for an athlete who has suffered little leaguer's elbow.

2. Develop a range of motion and strength program for an athlete who has suffered a posterior elbow dislocation.

I. Anatomy

Refer to Table 11-1 on page 421 in the text

II. Key Terms

Carrying angle — — — — The angle between the humerus and the ulna when the arm is in anatomical position

Cubital valgus — — — — — Angle of an extended elbow that deviates toward the radial side more than 20 degrees

Cubital varus — — — — — Angle of an extended elbow that deviates less than 10 degrees toward the radial side

Resting position — — — — Slightly flexed position of the elbow that allows for maximal volume to accommodate any intraarticular swelling

Volkmann's contracture— Ischemic necrosis of the forearm muscles and tissues caused by damage to the blood flow

Nightstick fracture — — — Fracture of the ulna due to a direct blow commonly seen in football players

Tackler's exostosis — — — Irritative exostosis arising from the anterior or lateral humerus

Ectopic bone — — — — — Proliferation of bone ossification in an abnormal place

Periostitis — — — — — — Inflammation of the periosteum (outer membrane covering the bone)

Fibrositis — — — — — — — Inflammation of fibrous tissue

Forearm splints — — — — Chronic strain to the forearm muscles

Epicondylitis — — — — — Inflammation and microrupturing of the soft tissues on the epicondyle of the distal humerus

Little leaguer's elbow — — Tension stress injury of the medial epicondyle seen in adolescents

Pronator syndrome — — — Median nerve is entrapped by the pronator teres, leading to pain on activities involving pronation

II. Key Terms (Con't)

Wrist drop — — — — — — Weakness and/or paralysis of the wrist and finger extensors due to damage to the radial nerve

Malaise — — — — — — — Lethargic feeling of general discomfort; out-of-sorts feeling

III. Kinematics

Refer to Table 11-1 on page 421 in the text and page 444 in the text.

Movement	Muscles	Normal ROM
Elbow flexion	Biceps brachii	140–150°
	Brachioradialis	
	Brachialis	
Elbow extension	Triceps brachii	0–10°
Forearm supination	Supinator	90°
Forearm pronation	Pronator quadratus	90°

IV. Simulations

 Lateral Epicondylitis (Tennis Elbow)

(Refer to pages 433–436 in the text)

During palpations, did you palpate the following structures for point tenderness, swelling, deformity, skin temperature, sensation, or other signs of trauma? Did you compare bilaterally?
- olecranon process
- radius
- ulna
- lateral epicondyle region
- proximal attachment of wrist extensor and supinator muscle groups

1A. During special tests, did you:
- perform active, passive, and resistive elbow flexion, extension, forearm supination and pronation, and wrist extension and flexion
- pay particular attention to manual resistance of wrist extension and supination, noting pain or tenderness near the lateral epicondyle
- ask the individual to squeeze each hand, comparing grip strength
- perform all tests bilaterally

Did your treatment protocol include ice, compression, elevation, anti-inflammatories, decrease in activities that aggravate the condition, and medical referral dependent on the degree of injury? (Refer to Field Strategy 11-5 on text page 437 for management protocol)

(Refer to pages 425–430 in the text)

Did you observe bilaterally for:
- swelling, discoloration, deformity, or other signs of trauma

Did you palpate bilaterally for:
- point tenderness, swelling, deformity, skin temperature, sensation, or other signs of trauma

2A. Did you suspect a contusion from the repetitive blocking activity of the football player? Since palpation revealed a hardend mass of soft tissue, did you suspect development of myositis ossificans? Treatment involves standard acute injury care and referral to a physician.

 3 Medial Epicondylitis "Little Leaguer's Elbow"

Refer to Field Strategy 11-4 on page 435 in the text.

During the history, did you determine if the injury was chronic or acute?
Did they ask:
- when, where, and how questions
- about throwing technique and training regimen (increase or decrease in throwing)
- what phase of the throwing motion pain occurs
- any previous injury, treatment, and medications
- the type of pain (dull, sharp, radiating, constant, intermittent, localized, general, increased during activity)
- ask if rest relieves symptoms

3A. Did you palpate the following structures bilaterally for point tenderness, swelling, deformity, sensation, skin temperature, or other signs of trauma?
- medial epicondyle
- origin of wrist flexors and pronators
- ulna
- olecranon
- ulnar nerve
- radius

During special tests, did you perform the following bilaterally?
- active, passive, and resisted elbow flexion, extension, forearm pronation and supination, and wrist extension and flexion
- pay particular attention to manual resistance of wrist flexion and pronation, noting pain or tenderness near the medial epicondyle
- ask the athlete to squeeze each hand, comparing grip strength
- perform Tinel's sign for ulnar nerve involvement

Did you determine that the ulnar nerve may be associated with this injury? Did you suspect medial epicondylitis or little leaguer's elbow?

V. Situations

l. Volkmann's Contracture - (Refer to page 439 in the text) - A major complication that results from a supracondylar fracture is Volkmann's contracture. Did you do the following to assess this condition?
- determine if the brachial artery or median nerve was damaged secondary to the fracture by looking and feeling for coldness, whiteness, or numbness in the hand of the affected arm
- perform passive extension of the fingers on the affected arm, noting increasing pain and aggravation to the injury

2. Forearm Fracture - Refer to Field Strategy 11-6 on page 441 in the text - To rule out injury to neurovascular structures of the forearm secondary to the forearm fracture, did you perform the following bilaterally:
- palpate for a distal radial or ulnar pulse
- check for sensation distal to the injury (See Figure 11-22 on page 448 in text)
- check for skin color and skin temperature distal to the injury

3. Olecranon Bursitis - (Refer to page 430 in the text)
- Did you identify this injury as olecranon bursitis?
- Did management include applying ice, compression, elevation, and other standard acute care procedures?

V. Situations (Con't)

4. Posterior Elbow Dislocation - (Refer to Field Strategy 11-2 on page 432 in the text) - To perform neurological and circulatory assessment for this injury, did you perform the following bilaterally?
- check for a distal pulse
- check for sensation distal to the injury
- check for skin color and skin temperature distal to the injury

Did you perform the following immediate first-aid care?
- immobilize the limb in position found
- treat for shock
- immediately refer to a physician or call 9ll for assistance

5. Compartment Syndrome - (Refer to page 438 in the text)
- Did you suspect a possible compartment syndrome?
- Did you determine that the following structures may be involved with this injury?
  - wrist and finger flexors of the anterior compartment
  - median nerve

VI. Special Tests to

Refer to pages 444 to 450 in the text.

VII. Multiple Choice Answers

l. b	8. b	15. b
2. d	9. a	16. b
3. c	10. b	17. a
4. a	11. d	18. c
5. b	12. a	19. b
6. d	13. c	20. d
7. a	14. d	

Chapter 12 — Wrist and Hand Injuries

After completing this chapter you should be able to:

• Locate the important bony and soft tissue structures of the wrist and hand

• Describe the motions of the wrist and hand and identify the muscles that produce them

• Explain what forces produce the loading patterns responsible for common injuries of the wrist and hand

• Recognize and manage common injuries to the wrist and hand

• Demonstrate a thorough assessment of the wrist and hand

• Demonstrate general rehabilitation exercises for the wrist and hand

I. Anatomy Review

Materials Needed:

SKELETON   ANATOMICAL WRIST AND HAND CHARTS   NONPERMANENT MARKERS

Instructions: *Work with a partner to perform the following:*
  - identify the following anatomical structures on the skeleton or anatomical charts
  - palpate and draw the anatomical structures on your partner using the nonpermanent marker.

────────────── Bony and Ligamentous Structures of the Wrist ──────────────

-radius
-ulna
-styloid process of ulna
-scaphoid or navicular
-lunate
-triquetrum
-pisiform
-trapezium

-trapezoid
-capitate
-hamate
-volar radiocarpal ligament
-dorsal radiocarpal ligament
-radial collateral ligament
-ulnar collateral ligament

Bony and Ligamentous Structures of the Hand and Fingers

-carpometacarpal joint
-intermetacarpal joint
-metacarpophalangeal joint
-interphalangeal joint

-metacarpal bones 1-5
-phalanges 1-5
-ulnar and radial collateral ligaments of
  thumb and phalanges

Muscles of the Wrist and Hand

-extensor pollicis longus
-extensor pollicis brevis
-flexor pollicis longus
-abductor pollicis longus
-extensor indicis
-extensor digitorum
-extensor digiti minimi
-flexor digitorum profundus
-flexor digitorum superficialis
-flexor pollicis brevis

-abductor pollicis brevis
-opponens pollicis
-adductor pollicis
-abductor digiti minimi
-flexor digiti minimi brevis
-opponens digiti minimi
-dorsal interossei
-palmar interossei
-lumbricales

Nerves and Blood Vessels of the Wrist and Hand

-median nerve
-ulnar nerve
-radial nerves

-radial artery
-ulnar artery
-digital arteries

II. Key Terms

Instructions: *Define the following terms.*

Volar
Dorsal
Saddle joint
Extrinsic muscles
Intrinsic muscles
Brachial plexus
Circumduction
Aseptic necrosis
Anatomical snuff box
Hypothenar

Thenar
Boxer's fracture
Bennett's fracture
Gamekeeper's thumb
Coach's finger
Jersey finger
Mallet finger
Boutonniere deformity
Trigger finger

de Quervain's tenosynovitis
Ganglion cyst
Subungual hematoma
Paronychia
Felon
Osteomyelitis
Carpal tunnel syndrome
Cyclist's palsy
Bowler's thumb

III. Kinematics of the Wrist and Hand

Instructions: *Work with a partner to perform the following. Have your partner perform the following movements while you name the muscles that are performing the movements along with the normal range of motion for each movement.* **(Refer to pages 459–462 and 484 in the text)**

	__Muscle__	__Range of Motion__
- forearm pronation and supination		
- wrist flexion and extension		
- radial deviation		
- ulnar deviation		
- finger flexion and extension		
- finger abduction and adduction		
- thumb flexion, extension, abduction, and adduction		
- opposition of the thumb and little finger		

Now that you have determined range of motion of the wrist and hand through subjective means, measure wrist and finger flexion with the use of a goniometer.

IV. Simulations

Instructions: *Perform the following simulated experiences.*

A cheerleader is complaining of pain over the right anatomical snuff box. Complete a history and observation of this injury.

1A. You have determined that the cheerleader fell on an outstretched hand yesterday during the execution of a back flip. Observation reveals minor swelling but no discoloration or deformity. Palpation reveals sharp pain in the anatomical snuff box. What injury should be suspected? How will you manage this injury?

The goalie on the soccer team reports a history of a hyperextension type injury to the ring finger of the right hand. Explain and demonstrate observation and palpation for this injury.

2A. Observation reveals minor swelling, some discoloration, but no deformity. Palpation produces point tenderness around the proximal phalanx that increases with compression and percussion along the long axis of the extended finger. You suspect a possible phalangeal fracture. Explain and demonstrate how to splint this type of fracture.

A gymnast is experiencing pain during vaulting and floor routines when the body weight is supported on the hands. Explain and demonstrate how to determine the difference between a wrist fracture and wrist sprain.

3A. All fracture tests are negative, and you believe the injury is a wrist sprain due to excessive extension. How will you manage this condition? Can the individual continue to practice with some support provided to prevent the injury from getting worse?

While holding a jersey tightly in one hand in an effort to stop the opposing player, a rugby player felt a sharp pain in the ring finger. Through observation and special tests, explain and demonstrate how to determine the differences between jersey finger and mallet finger. Identify what anatomical structures are involved with each injury.

4A. The observation and special tests conclude that the rugby player has ruptured the flexor digitorium profundus tendon of the injured finger. Explain and demonstrate the first-aid care for this injury.

V. Situations

Instructions: *Work with a partner to cooperatively analyze and address the following situations.*

1. A softball catcher was hit in the throwing hand by the bat of the hitter. Observation reveals immediate swelling over the fifth metacarpal of the affected hand. Explain and demonstrate how to determine a possible fracture, and then demonstrate how to properly immobilize the region and apply standard first-aid procedures.

2. A track athlete hit a hurdle and fell onto the cinder track and now has an abrasion on the palmar side of the hand. What immediate and long-term concerns must be kept in mind in cleaning this superficial wound?

3. An offensive lineman comes off the field complaining of pain in the right thumb. Explain and demonstrate how to determine the difference between a possible navicular fracture, ligament, and muscle injury.

4. A weight lifter pinched a finger between a weight and a weight rack. Blood has accumulated under the fingernail. The fingertip is extremely painful from the increasing pressure. What factors determine whether or not it is necessary to relieve the pressure?

V. Situations (Con't)

5. A long-distance cyclist is complaining of numbness in the little finger and medial half of the ring finger and is unable to abduct the little finger on both hands. The cyclist cannot recall a single incident that could have caused this condition. The cyclist's training distance has increased significantly in the past two weeks. What possible factors could be involved in this condition? What suggestions can be offered to help alleviate the symptoms yet allow the cyclist to continue training?

VI. Special Tests

Instructions: *Work with a partner to explain and demonstrate the following special tests:*

-Phalen's test   -Tinel's sign   -Froment's sign

VII. Multiple Choice Questions

Instructions: Choose the best answer for each question.

___1.   Most wrist motion occurs at the:
         a. radiocarpal joint   c. ulnar-radial joint
         b. ulnacarpal joint   d. carpalmetacarpal joint

___2.   The closed packed position of the proximal interphalangeal joint and the distal interphalangeal joints is:
         a. full flexion   c. opposition
         b. full extension   d. 20 degrees flexion

___3.   The flexors of the wrist and hand are innervated by the _____ nerve.
         a. ulna   c. musculocutaneous
         b. radial   d. median

___4.   The _____ nerve supplies afferent nerve supply to the fifth and half of the fourth finger on both the dorsal and palmar sides.
         a. ulna   c. musculocutaneous
         b. radial   d. median

___5.   The _____ artery is superficial and palpable on the anterior aspect of the wrist.
         a. ulnar   c. brachial
         b. radial   d. anterior interosseous artery

___6.   In what position should the wrist be held if maximum grip strength is desired?
         a. wrist in position of radial deviation and slight hyperextension
         b. wrist in position of ulnar deviation and slight hyperextension
         c. wrist in position of radial deviation and flexion
         d. wrist in position of ulnar deviation and flexion

___7. _____ is the mechanism of injury that is most often associated with fractures and dislocations at the distal forearm, wrist, and hand.
a. falling on an outstretched hand
b. falling on the apex of the elbow
c. direct blow
d. falling on the dorsal surface of the hand

___8. Gloves used in cycling, rowing, and weight lifting are used to:
a. decrease direct compression forces
b. decrease friction to the dorsal surface
c. cushion the dorsum of the hand
d. add padding to the palmar surface

___9. To strengthen the flexor muscles of the hand and wrist during rehabilitation, you could have the athlete perform:
a. bicep curls
b. rod and weight exercises
c. tennis ball squeezes
d. hammer exercises

___10. Infection can occur with hand abrasions. Which of these signs is not associated with an infection of an open wound to the hand?
a. tenderness
b. redness
c. deformity
d. swelling

___11. Most wrist injuries are caused by _____ on the proximal palm as a result of falling on an outstretched hand.
a. shear forces
b. axial loading
c. tensile forces
d. hyperradial deviation

___12. _____ is often a term used when the ulnar collateral ligament at the metacarpalphalangeal joint is torn during thumb hyperextension.
a. Colles' fracture
b. bowler's thumb
c. gamekeeper's thumb
d. jersey finger

___13. When the proximal phalanx is overstretched, injury to the _____ on the palmar side of the joint should be suspected.
a. volar plate
b. radial collateral ligament
c. ulnar collateral ligament
d. profundus

___14. Dislocations at the _____ are the most common hand joint dislocations.
a. distal interphalangeal joint
b. proximal interphalangeal joint
c. metacarpophalangeal joint
d. radial-ulnar joint

___15. Dislocations of the proximal interphalangeal joint should be splinted in:
a. 30 degrees of flexion
b. 30 degrees of extension
c. neutral position
d. slight hyperextension

___16. Avulsion of the extensor tendon from the attachment of the distal phalanx is termed:
a. jersey finger
b. mallet finger
c. trigger finger
d. bowler's thumb

___17. De Quervain's tenosynovitis exhibits pain during _____. The test used for De Quervain's tenosynovitis is _____.
a. wrist flexion, Phalen's
b. wrist extension, Phalen's
c. ulnar deviation, Finkelstein's
d. radial deviation, Finkelstein's

___18.   _____ strength is often limited during carpal tunnel syndrome.
a. extension   c. grip and pinch
b. extensor pollicis longus   d. radial deviation

___19.   An individual who complains of numbness in the little finger and who is unable to grasp a piece of paper between the thumb and index finger may have:
a. cyclist's palsy   c. carpal tunnel syndrome
b. De Quervain's tenosynovitis   d. ulnar neuropathy

___20.   Because of the poor blood supply to the anatomical snuff box, _____ is a common complication of a scaphoid fracture.
a. aseptic necrosis   c. lunate dislocation
b. Smith's fracture   d. neurological deficits

VIII. Additional Activities

1. **Visit an occupational therapist and have the therapist discuss and demonstrate exercises used in hand and wrist therapy.**

2. **Design a rehabilitation program for an athlete who has sustained a hyperextension wrist strain.**

3. **Design a strength program for a tennis player who wants to increase grip strength.**

I. Anatomy

Refer to Table 12-1 on pages 459–460 in the text.

II. Key Terms

Anatomical snuff box — — Region directly over the scaphoid bone bounded by the extensor pollicis brevis medially and the extensor pollicis longus laterally

Aseptic necrosis — — — — The death or decay of tissue due to a poor blood supply

Bennett's fracture — — — Fracture-dislocation to the proximal end of the first metacarpal at the carpal-metacarpal joint

Bowler's thumb — — — — Compression of the digital nerve on the medial aspect of the thumb, leading to paresthesia in the thumb

Boutonniere deformity — — Rupture of the central slip of the extensor tendon at the middle phalanx resulting in no active extensor mechanism at the PIP joint

Boxer's fracture — — — — Fracture of the fifth metacarpal, resulting in a flexion deformity due to rotation of the head of the metacarpal over the neck

Brachial plexus — — — — Nerve plexus formed by the intertwined ventral rami of the lower four cervical and first thoracic nerves (C_5-T_1)

Carpal tunnel syndrome — Compression of the median nerve as it passes through the carpal tunnel, leading to pain and tingling in the hand

Circumduction — — — — Circular motion of a body segment, resulting from sequential flexion, abduction, extension, and adduction, or vice versa

Coach's finger — — — — — Fixed flexion deformity of the finger, resulting from dislocation at the PIP joint

Colles' fracture — — — — Fracture involving a dorsally angulated and displaced, and a radially angulated and displaced fracture within one and one-half inches of the wrist

II. Key Terms (Con't)

Cyclist's palsy — — — — Seen when biker's lean on the handlebar an extended period of time resulting in paresthesia in the ulnar nerve distribution

de Quervain's tenosynovitis· An inflammatory stenosing tenosynovitis of the abductor pollicis longus and extensor pollicis brevis tendons

Dorsal — — — — — — Referring to the back of the hand

Extrinsic muscles — — — Muscles with the proximal attachment located outside of the body part it moves or acts upon

Felon — — — — — — — Abscess within the fat pad of the fingertip

Galeazzi's fracture — — — Radial fracture with an associated dislocation of the ulna at the distal radial ulnar joint

Ganglion cyst — — — — Benign tumor mass commonly seen on the dorsal aspect of the wrist

Hypothenar — — — — — Mass of intrinsic muscles of the little finger, including the abductor digiti minimi, flexor digiti minimi brevis, and opponens digiti minimi

Intrinsic muscles — — — — Muscles with the proximal and distal attachments located within the body part it moves or acts upon

Jersey finger — — — — — Rupture of the flexor digitorum profundus tendon from the distal phalanx due to rapid extension of the finger while actively flexed

Mallet finger — — — — — Rupture of the extensor tendon from the distal phalanx due to forceful flexion of the phalanx

Monteggia's fracture — — Ulnar fracture with an associated dislocation of the radial head

Osteomyelitis — — — — — Inflammation or infection of the bone and bone marrow

Paronychia — — — — — — Infection along the nail fold commonly associated with a hangnail

II. Key Terms (Con't)

Saddle joint — — — — — Joint at which one bone surface has a concave saddle-like shape and the articulating bone surface is reciprocally shaped

Smith fracture — — — — Forearm fracture with volar angulation or displacement; opposite of Colles' fracture

Stenosing — — — — — — Narrowing of an opening or stricture of a canal; stenosis

Subungual hematoma — — Collection of blood under the fingernail caused by direct trauma

Thenar — — — — — — — Mass of intrinsic muscles of the thumb including the flexor pollicis brevis, abductor pollicis brevis, and opponens pollicis

Trigger finger — — — — Condition whereby the finger flexors contract but are unable to reextend because of a nodule within the tendon sheath or the sheath being too constricted to allow free motion

Volar — — — — — — — Referring to the palm of the hand

III. Kinematics of the Wrist and Hand

Refer to Table 12-1 on pages 459–460 in the text and to page 484 in the text.

Motion	Muscles	Range of Motion
Wrist flexion	Flexor carpi radialis	80–90°
	Flexor carpi ulnaris	
	Palmaris longus	
Wrist extension	Extensor carpi radialis longus	70–90°
	Extensor carpi radialis brevis	
	Extensor carpi ulnaris	
Radial deviation	Flexor carpi radialis	15°
	Extensor carpi radialis	
Ulnar deviation	Flexor carpi ulnaris	30–45°
	Extensor carpi ulnaris	

IV. Simulations

 Scaphoid

Refer to page 477 to 478 in the text

During the history, did you ask:
- where, when, and how questions
- if the injury was acute or chronic
- about the type of pain the individual is experiencing (dull, sharp, radiating, constant, intermittent, localized, general, increased during activity)
- ask about previous injuries, treatment, or medications.
(Refer to Field Strategy 12-3 text page 481)

During observations, did you observe bilaterally for:
- swelling, discoloration, deformity, and other signs of trauma
- the shape, contour, and posture of the hand
- surgical scars or incisions

Did you palpate bilaterally for:
- swelling, temperature, deformity, point tenderness
- other signs of trauma

1A. Did you suspect a fracture to the scaphoid because of point tenderness over the anatomical snuff box?

 Phalangeal Fracture

Did you observe bilaterally for swelling, deformity, discoloration, or other signs of trauma?

Did you palpate bilaterally for point tenderness, swelling, crepitation, deformity, sensation, and circulation?

2A. Did you immobilize the injured finger in 30 degrees of flexion to reduce the pull of the flexor tendon?

(Refer to Field Strategies 12-3 on page 481 in the text and 12-4 on page 483 in the text).

To determine a possible wrist fracture, did you:
- determine the mechanism of injury in the history
- palpate for point tenderness and crepitus over the bones and observe for any deformity
- ask the individual to perform active range of motion to determine willingness and physiological functioning of the region
- perform compression, distraction, and percussion tests for a possible fracture

If fracture tests were negative, did you apply resisted range of motion exercises to determine a possible wrist sprain

3A. Did you manage the wrist sprain with:
- ice, compression, elevation,
- progressive range of motion and strength exercises
- supportive taping or bracing

Jersey Finger

(Refer to page 469 in the text)

Did you observe bilaterally for:
- swelling, deformity, discoloration, and other signs of trauma
- deformity of the distal attachment of the flexor profundus tendon
- the functioning of the flexor profundus tendon by asking the individual to actively flex the PIP joint while keeping the distal interphalangeal joint extended

Mallet Finger
- observe for deformity of the distal attachment of the extensor tendon
- test the function of the extensor tendon by asking the individual to actively extend the DIP joint of the effected finger

4A. Did you immobilize the affected finger, apply ice, and refer the person to a physician?

V. Situations

l. Metacarpal Fracture - (Refer to Field Strategy 12-2 on page 479 in the text) -
To determine if the injury is a possible fracture did you:
- perform a history to determine the mechanism of injury
- observe for swelling, discoloration, deformity, or bone protrusions
- palpate for deformity, crepitation, and point tenderness over the metacarpal area
- apply compression and percussion through the axis of the fifth metacarpal, noting increased pain

To care for this injury, did you:
- immobilize the hand in a relaxed fist position, apply ice, and refer to a physician

2. Abrasion - Immediate concerns for this abrasion injury include:
- preventing HIV or hepatitis B virus (HBV) by using universal precautions (Refer to pages 61 and 464 in text)
- cleansing the wound thoroughly to prevent infection
- applying sterile nonadherent dressing

Long-term concerns for this abrasion may include:
- checking the wound daily for signs of infection
- referring the individual to a physician if infection is noted

3. Thumb Injury - Did you determine that:
- a scaphoid fracture would produce pain over the anatomical snuff box and increase with radial deviation and wrist extension
- to test a ligament injury to the thumb, a valgus or varus stress test is applied to determine laxity of the ligaments if no fracture is suspected
- to determine a muscle injury, active and resistive range of motion can be applied to the thumb musculature

4. Subungual Hematoma - (Refer to Field Strategy 12-1 on page 473 in the text) -
Did you determine that the athlete has a subungual hematoma? Did you decide that if it is not absolutely necessary to relieve the pressure from under the nail, they should not do so because this opens an avenue for infection? If pressure must be relieved, the procedure should be carried out under the direction of a physician.

V. Situations (Con't)

5. Cyclist's Palsy - (Refer to text pages 475 to 476) - Did you determine the condition to be cyclist's palsy and that factors related to this condition include:
- leaning on the handlebar for extended period of time
- not switching hand positions frequently
- improper fit of the bike to the rider

Did you offer the following suggestions to help alleviate the symptoms so that the cyclist could continue training?
- padding the handlebars
- wearing padded gloves
- varying hand positions
- getting properly fitted for the bike

VI. Special Tests

Refer to pages 483 to 489 in the text

VII. Multiple Choice Answers

1. a	8. d	15. a
2. b	9. c	16. b
3. d	10. c	17. c
4. a	11. b	18. c
5. b	12. c	19. d
6. b	13. a	20. a
7. a	14. b	

Chapter 13 — Head and Facial Injuries

After completing this chapter you should be able to:

- Locate the important bony and soft tissue structures of the head and facial region

- Identify forces responsible for common injuries to the head and facial region

- Recognize specific injuries to the skull and facial area

- Demonstrate a thorough assessment of a cerebral injury

- Recognize and demonstrate immediate care of facial injuries

- Identify protective padding and commercial products used to prevent and manage head and facial injuries

I. Anatomy Review

Materials Needed:

SKELETON   ANATOMICAL CHARTS OF HEAD AND FACE   NONPERMANENT MARKERS

Instructions: *Work with a partner to perform the following:*
- *identify the following anatomical structures on the skeleton or anatomical charts.*
- *palpate and draw the anatomical structures on your partner using the nonpermanent marker.*

Structures of the Head and Face

-frontal bone
-occipital bone
-sphenoid bone
-ethmoid bone
-parietal bone
-temporal bone
-maxilla
-mandible

-zygomatic arch
-nasal bone
-lacrimal
-glabella
-palatine
-temporal mandibular joint
-carotid artery
-cranial nerves

Identify the functions of the following anatomical structures:

-optic nerve
-olfactory nerve
-oculomotor and trochlear nerves
-vestibulocochlear nerve
-gray matter of cerebral cortex
-medulla oblongata

-cerebrum
-cerebellum
-lacrimal glands
-iris
-retina
-middle meningeal artery

II. Key Terms

Instructions: *Define the following terms.*

Dyspnea
Tinnitus
Cauliflower ear
Vertigo
Photophobia
Battle's sign
Concussion
Postconcussion syndrome
Post-traumatic memory loss
Retrograde amnesia
Diffuse injuries
Dural sinuses
Focal injuries

Meninges
Meningitis
Gray matter
White matter
Epistaxis
Malocclusion
Intruded
Extruded
Otitis media
Otitis externa
Serous otitis
Conjunctivitis

Sty
Subconjunctival hemorrhage
Tunics
Hyphema
Diplopia
Myopia
Detached retina
Nystagmus
Periorbital ecchymosis
Raccoon eyes
Contrecoup injuries
Decompression

III. Simulations and Situations

Instructions: *Perform the following simulated experiences.*

l. A basketball player has fallen and sustained what appears to be a superficial cut on the back of the head. The cut is bleeding profusely. What anatomical structure(s) are likely to have been damaged and why? How serious is this injury likely to be? Explain and demonstrate the immediate treatment protocol.

2. A rugby player was hit in the torso region and is down on the field. During the history, you learn that the neck is sore and the player has a headache, and is also a bit dazed and dizzy. This information is confusing because you saw the injury and know that the player did not receive a blow to the head. Explain how and why the individual may be experiencing these symptoms. What other signs and symptoms should be farther investigated during the HOPS process? How would you determine when this individual should return to participation?

III. Simulations and Situations (Con't)

3. A softball player collided with the shortstop, accidentally taking an elbow to the side of the head. The individual is dizzy and has a mild headache. There is no immediate memory loss, and the pupils are normal. After 15 minutes of icing the injured area, the individual reports an increasing headache and is feeling nauseous. The player appears lethargic, disoriented, and sensitive to sunlight. What might be happening, and how will you manage this situation?

4. A swimmer during a backstroke set misjudged the distance to the wall and collided head first into the wall. After the assessment, you determine the swimmer experienced a mild concussion. What instructions are you going to give the swimmer when leaving for the day? What follow-up care will you provide?

4A. Two days after the swimmer experienced the injury, he/she reports a persistent headache and an inability to concentrate. What other questions should be asked of the swimmer about the condition? What condition may the swimmer be experiencing? What is standard protocol for managing this injury?

5. A hockey player was taking a shot on goal when the stick hit the jaw of the player who was guarding him. That player came off the ice bleeding from the mouth and unable to close the jaw. Explain and demonstrate observation and palpation of this hockey player. What type of injury do you suspect and why?

6. In fielding a softball, the third baseman was struck in the nose by the ball. Explain and demonstrate how to determine the difference between an epistaxis and possible nasal fracture through the evaluation procedures. What treatment protocol would be used for each injury?

7. A basketball player was going up for a rebound and was struck in the eye by an opposing player's finger. The eye is swollen and closed. Attempts to open the eye causes tearing and pain. Explain and demonstrate how to determine the differences between a periorbital ecchymosis, corneal abrasion, detached retina, and possible orbital fracture. Explain the treatment protocol for each condition.

IV. Special Test

Instructions: *Work with a partner to perform the following special tests and explain the rationale for each test.*

- 100 minus 7 test
- Romberg's test
- Heel/toe walking

- Finger to nose test
- Stork stand

V. Multiple Choice Questions

Instructions: *Choose the best answer for each question.*

___1. The immovable joints of the skull are referred to as:
 a. sutures
 b. bridges
 c. the cranium
 d. palatines

___2. The scalp and face tend to bleed profusely upon laceration because of their
 a. avascular properties
 b. vascular properties
 c. dense tissue
 d. subcutaneous tissue

___3. The ____ portion of the brain is responsible for motor and sensory function.
 a. brain stem
 b. white matter
 c. gray matter
 d. diencephalon

___4. The ____ controls the size of the pupil, regulating the amount of light that enters the eye.
 a. sclera
 b. tunic
 c. iris
 d. lacrimal

___5. The olfactory nerve has _____ functions.
 a. motor
 b. sensory
 c. reflexive
 d. accessory

___6. The most important preventative measure for head and facial injuries is:
 a. protective equipment
 b. conditioning
 c. proper skill technique
 d. preseason physical

___7. Mechanical failure of a bone such as in a fractured mandible usually occurs from an overload of:
 a. compression
 b. chronic stress
 c. shearing force
 d. tensile stress

___8. ____ injuries may only account for one-quarter of the fatalities due to head trauma, but they are the most prevalent cause of long-term neurological deficits.
 a. focal
 b. diffuse
 c. compression
 d. deceleration

___9. An athlete has received a blow to the head, and discoloration is occurring behind an ear of the athlete. What injury do you suspect?
 a. contrecoup concussion
 b. meningitis
 c. subdural hematoma
 d. basilar fracture

___10. If after a blow to the head an athlete appears fine but within 10 to 20 minutes starts to exhibit signs and symptoms of neurological deterioration, such as drowsiness, nausea, vomiting, and decreased level of consciousness, what injury should you suspect?
 a. basilar fracture
 b. concussion
 c. subdural hematoma
 d. epidural hematoma

___11. Concussions are graded by:
 a. the length of mental impairment
 b. the loss of memory before and after injury
 c. the force
 d. the length of mental impairment and loss of memory before and after injury

___12. Asking the athlete how they got to the game, what quarter they were injured, and what day of the week it is after a head injury is testing the athlete's:

    a. retrograde memory   c. mental acuity

    b. post-traumatic memory   d. level of consciousness

___13. When caring for an unconscious athlete never:

    a. collect a history from witnesses

    b. place ammonia capsules under the nose to arouse the athlete

    c. stabilize the head and neck

    d. check vital signs

___14. The Glasgow Coma Scale is used to determine an individual's:

    a. rate of breathing   c. auditory functioning

    b. response to stimulation   d. olfactory functioning

___15. Abnormal facial expression and functioning may indicate:

    a. concussion   c. cerebral damage

    b. brain stem damage   d. loss of sensory functions

___16. After sustaining a head injury, an athlete's skin becomes pale and clammy. What might you suspect is occurring?

    a. heat stroke   c. shock

    b. heat exhaustion   d. obstructed airway

___17. To determine an individual's balance after sustaining a head injury you would have the athlete perform:

    a. the 100 minus 7 test   c. the six cardinal planes of vision test

    b. shoulder shrug test   d. the stork stand test

___18. If after being hit in the face, an athlete's cheek appears flat or depressed with swelling about the eye, you should suspect:

    a. zygomatic arch fracture   c. temporomandibular dislocation

    b. maxillary fracture   d. dislocated mandible

___19. Signs of a _____ should always be checked with a nasal fracture because of the nasal bones proximity to the cranial region.

    a. basilar fracture   c. epidural hematoma

    b. concussion   d. maxillary fracture

___20. After sustaining an eye injury, an athlete reports seeing floaters or lights flashing. What eye injury should you suspect?

    a. detached retina   c. corneal abrasion

    b. orbital fracture   d. hyphema

VI. Additional Activities

1. **Visit with an opthamologist and dentist to further discuss eye and oral injuries associated with sports.**

2. **Evaluate your school's sports program to determine if it is providing protective measures in preventing head and facial injuries.**

3. **Fit a football helmet to specifications to prevent head and facial injuries.**

4. **Evaluate your athletic training kit to make sure you have supplies and equipment needed to treat head and facial injuries if they were to occur.**

Student's Key

I. Anatomy

Refer to Figure 13-1 on page 498 in the text and Table 13-1 on page 501 in the text.

II. Key Terms

Dyspnea — — — — — — — Shortness of breath or difficulty in breathing

Tinnitus — — — — — — — Ringing or other noises in the ear due to trauma or disease

Cauliflower ear — — — — Hematoma between the perichondrium and cartilage of the outer ear; auricular hematoma

Vertigo — — — — — — — Balance disturbance characterized by a whirling sensation of one's self or external objects

Photophobia — — — — — Abnormal sensitivity to light

Battle's sign — — — — — Delayed discoloration behind the ear due to basilar skull fracture

Concussion — — — — — — Violent shaking or jarring action of the brain, resulting in immediate or transient impairment of neurological function

Postconcussion syndrome — Delayed condition characterized by persistent headaches, blurred vision, irritability, and inability to concentrate

Post-traumatic memory loss — Forgetting events after an injury

Retrograde amnesia — — — Forgetting events prior to an injury

Diffuse injuries — — — — Widespread disruption to the function and/or structure of the brain

Dural sinuses — — — — — Formed by tubular separations in the inner and outer layers of the dura matter, these sinuses function as small veins for the brain

Focal injuries — — — — — Localized cerebral damage

Meninges — — — — — — Three protective membranes that surround the brain and spinal cord

II. Key Terms (Con't)

Meningitis — — — — — Inflammation of the meninges of the brain and spinal column

Gray matter — — — — Composed of neuron cell bodies, dendrites, and short unmyelinated axons

White matter — — — — Composed of myelinated nerve axons; it is the myelin sheaths that give the tissue its characteristic white coloring

Epistaxis — — — — — — Profuse bleeding from the nose

Malocclusion — — — — Inability to bring teeth together in a normal bite

Intruded — — — — — — Tooth driven in an inward direction

Extruded — — — — — Tooth driven in an outward direction

Otitis media — — — — Localized infection in the middle ear secondary to upper respiratory infections

Otitis externa — — — — Bacterial infection involving the lining of the auditory canal; swimmer's ear

Serous otitis — — — — Fluid buildup behind the eardrum in association with otitis media and upper respiratory infections

Conjunctivitis — — — — Bacterial infection leading to itching, burning, watering, inflamed eye; pinkeye

Sty — — — — — — — — Infection of the sebaceous gland of an eyelash or eyelash follicle

Subconjunctival hemorrhage- Minor capillary ruptures in the eye globe

Tunics — — — — — — Three layers of protective tissues that surround the eye

Hyphema — — — — — Serious condition with hemorrhage into the anterior chamber of the eye

Diplopia — — — — — — Double vision

Myopia — — — — — — Nearsightedness

II. Key Terms (Con't)

Detached retina — — — — Neurosensory retina is separated from the retinal epithelium by swelling

Nystagmus — — — — — — Abnormal jerking or involuntary eye movement

Periorbital ecchymosis — — Swelling and hemorrhage into the surrounding eye lids; black eye

Raccoon eyes — — — — — Delayed discoloration around the eyes from anterior cranial fossa fracture

Contrecoup injuries — — — Injuries away from the actual injury site due to axial rotation and acceleration

Decompression — — — — Surgical release of pressure from fluid or blood accumulation

III. Simulations and Situations

l. Scalp Laceration - Refer to page 512 in the text - Did you evaluate the athlete for a possible concussion? Did you use universal precautions during your evaluation and treatment protocol? Did you apply direct pressure to the wound, bandage, and ice? Did you refer the basketball player to a physician for possible sutures?

2. Concussion - Refer to pages 509 to 512 and Tables 13-4 (text page 511) and 13-6 (text page 519) - Did you determine that the rugby player may have a contre-coup concussion? Did you further evaluate the rugby player by performing a HOPS assessment for a concussion? Did you determine if the player could return to activity according to the signs and symptoms presented, particularly to those related to con-sciousness and memory loss?

3. Severe Concussion/Head Injury - Did you determine that an immediate physician referral was needed since the softball player may be experiencing signs and symp-toms related to a possible epidural hematoma?

4. Postconcussion Syndrome - Did you determine that the swimmer may be experi-encing postconcussion syndrome? Did you further investigate the swimmer's condi-tion by asking further questions related to postconcussion syndrome? Did you refer the swimmer to a physician?

(Refer to Field Strategy 13-2 on page 518 in the text and Table 13-6 on page 519 in the text for further identification and treatment procedures for cranial injuries)

III. Simulations and Situations (Con't)

5. Fractured Mandible - Did you observe the following?
- malocclusion
- deformity
- swelling
- other signs of trauma (lacerations)

Did you palpate the following structures for point tenderness, muscle spasms, and deformity?
- maxilla
- mandible
- zygomatic
- nasal bone
- temporal mandibular joint (TMJ)
- other related soft tissue

Did you practice universal precautions since the individual was bleeding from the mouth?

Did you conclude that the hockey player may have a fractured mandible? What is the treatment protocol for this injury? (Refer to text pages 519 to 520)

6. Nasal Injury - Refer to text pages 521 to 523 and Field Strategy 13-4 on page 524. - Did you explain and demonstrate that a nasal fracture would indicate the following signs?
- deformity
- swelling
- crepitus in the bridge of the nasion
- ecchymosis under the eyes

Did you stand behind and above the injured player to observe the injury? What protocol would be used for a nasal fracture and epistaxis?

III. Simulations and Situations (Con't)

7. Eye Injury - Refer to text pages 527 to 530 and Field Strategy 13-6 on pages 532. - Did you conclude that a corneal abrasion may be present because of the:
- tearing
- pain upon movement
- increased pain upon blinking of eye
- photophobia

Did you determine that a detached retina would result in lights flashing on and off when the individual opened the eyes several days following the injury, or they might state that a blanket has covered part of the field of vision?

During your assessment of an orbital fracture, did you ask the athlete to look upward with both eyes and observe if the injured eye failed to do this movement?

How did you indicate you would treat each of these eye injuries? In each case, what would determine a physician referral? (Refer to Field Strategy 13-6 on page 532 in the text)

IV. Special Tests

Refer to pages 513–516 in the text

V. Multiple Choice Answers

l. a	8. b	15. c
2. b	9. d	16. c
3. c	10. d	17. d
4. c	11. d	18. a
5. b	12. a	19. b
6. a	13. b	20. a
7. d	14. b	

Chapter 14 — Injuries to the Spine

After completing this chapter you should be able to:

• Locate and explain the functional significance of the important bony and soft tissue structures of the spine

• Describe the motion capabilities in the different regions of the spine

• Explain what factors contribute to mechanical loads on the spine

• Specify strategies to reduce spinal stress in preventing low back pain

• Identify anatomical variations that may predispose individuals to spine injuries

• Recognize and describe common sports injuries to the spine and back

• Demonstrate a thorough assessment of the spine

• Demonstrate rehabilitative exercises for the spine

I. Anatomy Review

Materials Needed:

SKELETON   ANATOMICAL SPINE CHARTS   NONPERMANENT MARKERS

Instructions: *Work with a partner to perform the following.*
 - *identify the following anatomical structures on the skeleton or anatomical charts*
 - *palpate and draw the anatomical structures on your partner using the nonpermanent marker.*

Structures of the Spine

-cervical spines Cl-C7
-thoracic spines Tl-T12
-lumbar spines L1-L5
-sacral spines Sl-S5
-coccyx
-intervertebral disc
-pars articularis
-spinous and transverse process
-axis and atlas
-supraspinous ligament
-ligament flavum

-sternocleidomastoid
-trapezius
-erector spinae
-levator scapula
-occiput
-mastoid process
-lumbar curve
-cervical curve
-thoracic curve
-cauda equina

II. Key Terms

Define the following terms.

Motion segment
Atlas
Axis
Annulus fibrous
Nucleus pulposus
Cauda equina
Reflex
Kyphosis

Lordosis
Scheuermann's disease
Scoliosis
Spondylolisthesis
Spondylolysis
Spina bifida occulata
Spinal stenosis
Neurapraxia

Burner
Wedged fracture
Osteopenia
Sciatica
Prolapsed disc
Extruded disc
Coccygodynia
Ipsilateral

III. Kinematics

Instructions: *Work with a partner to perform the following:*

1. Have your partner perform spinal flexion and extension. In what plane of movement are the motions occurring? Does maximal spinal flexion and extension occur in the lumbar, cervical, or thoracic vertebra? What is the degree of maximal spinal flexion?

2. Have your partner perform lateral flexion. In what plane of movement does this motion occur? What is the normal degree of motion for lateral flexion in the lumbar vertebra?

3. Have your partner perform spinal rotation and forward bending of the cervical vertebra. What is the average range of motion for cervical rotation and forward bending?

IV. Simulations

Instructions: *Perform the following simulated experiences.*

A football player is down on the field and you have been beckoned to render care. The individual is lying supine, the head turned to the side, and he is not moving. Perform a primary assessment.

1A. The athlete has a pulse and is breathing adequately. The individual has regained consciousness. Continue with the secondary survey and conduct a history of this injury. Would you remove the face mask on the athlete?

1B. During the history you discover the player is dizzy, has a mild headache and has mild pain in the neck. Explain and demonstrate observation, palpation, and special testing procedures.

IC. After completing the on-the-field secondary survey, the player still has a mild headache, mild neck pain, and is somewhat dizzy, but complete sensory and motor function appears normal. Explain and demonstrate how to remove the player from the field. Explain and demonstrate a full off-the-field assessment for this injury.

ID. You have rechecked the player's balance, neck range of motion, vital signs, vision, memory, and have reevaluated for concussion. What criteria will determine if the player can return to competition or must be immediately transported to the hospital?

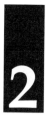

A defensive lineman charged the quarterback preparing to throw a pass and struck the throwing arm, forcing it into excessive external rotation, abduction, and extension. An immediate burning sensation traveled down the length of the quarterback's arm, and now his thumb is tingling. What might have happened here? Explain and demonstrate your observations and palpations. What special tests would you use?

2A. The quarterback exhibits radiating pain down his right arm into his thumb, and he has weakness in his biceps. The tingling resolves within a few minutes. What criteria are used to determine when the player can return to participation?

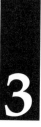

A cheerleader is complaining of an aching pain during trunk flexion aggravated with resisted hyperextension that produces sharp shooting pains into the low back and down the posterior leg. This condition has been present for four weeks and is not getting better. The individual cannot recall a traumatic episode that may have caused the condition. A physician has not been seen nor have radiographs been taken of the lumbar region. Explain and demonstrate palpation procedures for this injury.

3A. What special tests can rule out a disc injury? What special tests can identify if the injury is nerve related? Explain and demonstrate these tests.

3B. What criteria are used to determine if the individual should be referred to a physician?

V. Situations

Instructions: *Work with a partner to cooperatively analyze and answer the following situations.*

1. After practice, a wrestler is complaining of a sore neck that is most comfortable with the head in a slightly rotated position to the right. Point tenderness is present in the left sternocleidomastoid muscle and right trapezius muscle. Explain and demonstrate the special testing procedures for this injury. While doing these tests, please indicate the normal range of motion for the various neck movements.

2. An adolescent butterfly stroker is complaining of localized pain and tenderness in the midback region. The pain developed gradually and only hurts during execution of the stroke. Explain and demonstrate palpations and special tests using the HOPS procedure. During the assessment, perform a scan examination. What conditions would you suspect to occur in this area of the thoracic spine?

VI. Special Tests

Instructions: *Work with a partner to perform the following special tests and explain the rational for each test.*

- Myotome testing
- Cervical compression test
- Cervical distraction test
- Straight leg raising test
- Reflex testing
- Prone knee bending test
- Sacroiliac test

VII. Multiple Choice Questions

Instructions: *Choose the best answer for each question.*

___1. The _____ is the functional unit of the spine.
    a. vertebra   c. motion segment
    b. intervertebral disc   d. facets

___2. The region of the vertebrae is most susceptible to stress fractures.
    a. pars   c. neural arch
    b. posterior body   d. vertebral arch

___3. The limit range of motion in the different spinal regions.
    a. intervertebral disc   c. facet joints
    b. adjacent pedicle   d. transverse processes

___4. The thoracic and sacral curves of the spine are _____.
    a. convexed anteriorly   c. concaved anteriorly
    b. convexed posteriorly   d. concaved posteriorly

___5. When the spine is extended backward past anatomical position, the motion
is termed _____. This motion takes place in the _____ plane.
   a. extension, sagittal
   b. flexion, sagittal
   c. hyperextension, frontal
   d. hyperextension, sagittal

___6. Spinal rotation is greatest in the _____ region.
   a. cervical
   b. thoracic
   c. lumbar
   d. sacral

___7. When the body is in an upright position, the major form of loading of the spine is:
   a. shearing force
   b. tension force
   c. axial
   d. atlas

___8. Compression on the lumbar spine increases with:
   a. standing for prolonged periods of time
   b. lying flat
   c. sitting and spinal extension
   d. sitting and spinal flexion

___9. Lifting an object with _____ movements increases compression
and shearing forces on the spine.
   a. slow and intentional
   b. slow and jerky
   c. rapid and jerky
   d. intermittent

___10. Lifting with the trunk _____ minimizes the tension requirement for
muscles of the lumbar spine.
   a. extended
   b. rotated
   c. flexed
   d. erect

___11. Scheuermann's disease is associated with:
   a. lordosis
   b. kyphosis
   c. sway back
   d. scoliosis

___12. Spondylolysis often occurs because of:
   a. repeated axial loading of the lumbar spine when it is hyperextended
   b. repeated axial loading of the lumbar spine when it is hyperflexed
   c. repeated axial loading of the cervical spine when it is hyperflexed
   d. acute trauma to the lumbar and cervical spine

___13. During spondylolysis and spondylolisthesis, muscle spasms often occur in the:
   a. rectus abdominis
   b. erector spinae and hamstrings
   c. erector spinae and quadriceps
   d. external and internal obliques

___14. Flexibility and strengthening of the _____ muscles are imperative to
stabilization of the spine.
   a. abdominal
   b. pelvic
   c. back
   d. thigh

___15. Nerve root injuries are always _____ differentiating them from other motor
and sensory changes involved with spinal injuries.
   a. unilateral
   b. transient
   c. bilateral
   d. intermittent

___16. Cervical strains most often involve the:
   a. levator scapula
   b. sternocleidomastoid
   c. occiput
   d. lower trapezius

____17. During a brachial plexus injury, muscular weakness is evident in the:
   a. internal rotators and deltoid
   b. external rotators and deltoid
   c. external rotators, deltoid, and biceps brachii
   d. internal rotators, deltoid, and biceps brachii
____18. Runners are often at risk for low back pain due to:
   a. tight hip extensors and quadricep muscles
   b. tight hip flexors and hamstrings muscles
   c. tight abdominal muscles
   d. tight back muscles
____19. If nerve root L5 is irritated or damaged, myotome weakness will be found in:
   a. toe flexion
   b. toe extension
   c. ankle dorsiflexion
   d. ankle plantar flexion
____20. The Adam's position is used to determine:
   a. spinal flexion
   b. spinal extension
   c. spinal flexion and scoliosis
   d. spinal extension and scoliosis

VIII. Additional Activities

l. **Visit a radiologist and ask the radiologist to show you various types of x-rays of back conditions.**

2. **Visit a physical therapist and observe various low back rehabilitation programs and exercises.**

3. **Apply a neck roll and shoulder pads to a football player.**

4. **Demonstrate proper lifting techniques to decrease low back injury to a fellow classmate.**

I. Anatomy

Refer to Figures 14-1 and 14-2 text pages 536 to 537 and Table 14-1 on text pages 541 to 542.

II. Key Terms

Motion segment — — — — Two adjacent vertebrae and the intervening soft tissues; the functional unit of the spine

Atlas — — — — — — — The first cervical vertebra; named because it supports the skull

Axis — — — — — — — The second cervical vertebra; named after its bony prominence around which the atlas rotates

Annulus fibrous — — — — Tough outer covering of the intervertebral disc composed of fibrocartilage

Nucleus pulposus — — — — Gelatinous-like material comprising the inner portion of the intervertebral disc

Cauda equina — — — — — Lower spinal nerves that course through the lumbar spinal canal, resembling a horse's tail

Reflex — — — — — — — Action involving stimulation of a motor neuron by a sensory neuron in the spinal cord without involvement of the brain

Kyphosis — — — — — — Excessive curve in the thoracic region of the spine

Lordosis — — — — — — Excessive curve in the lumbar region of the spine

Scheuermann's disease — Osteochondrosis of the spine due to abnormal epiphyseal plate behavior that allows herniation of the disc into the vertebral body, giving a characteristic wedge-shaped appearance

Scoliosis — — — — — — Lateral rotational spinal curvature

Spondylolisthesis — — — — Anterior slippage of a vertebrae, resulting from a complete bilateral fracture of the pars interarticularis

Spondylolysis — — — — — A stress fracture of the pars interarticularis

II. Key Terms (Con't)

Spina bifida occulata — — Congenital defect in the vertebral canal characterized by absence of the laminae and spinous process

Spinal stenosis — — — — A loss of cerebrospinal fluid around the spinal cord due to deformation of the spinal cord or a narrowing of the neural canal

Neurapraxia — — — — Injury to a nerve that results in temporary neurological deficits followed by complete recovery of function

Burner — — — — — — Burning or stinging sensation characteristic of a brachial plexus injury

Wedged fracture — — — — A crushing compression fracture that leaves a vertebra narrowed anteriorly

Osteopoenia — — — — Condition of reduced bone mineralization or density of a bone

Sciatica — — — — — — Compression of a spinal nerve due to a herniated disc, annular tear, myogenic or muscle-related disease, spinal stenosis, facet joint arthropathy, or compression from the piriformis muscle

Prolapsed disc — — — — Condition when the eccentric nucleus produces a definite deformity as it works its way through the fibers of the annulus fibrous

Extruded disc — — — — Condition in which the nuclear material come into the spinal canal and runs the risk of impinging adjacent nerve roots

Coccygodynia — — — — Prolonged or chronic pain in the coccygeal region due to irritation of the coccygeal nerve plexus

Ipsilateral — — — — — Situated on, pertaining to, or affecting the same side, as opposed to contralateral

III. Kinematics

Cervical Spine
(Refer to pages 542 to 544 and Table 14-2 [text page 544])

IV. Simulations

 Head/Neck Down on the Field

Refer to pages 566 to 570 in the text

During the primary assessment, did you:
- check for consciousness by shouting the athlete's name?
- check for pulse by palpating the carotid artery?
- check for breathing by palpating or watching the chest rise and fall
- check the pupils for size and responsiveness
- An athlete's pulse rate will range from 40 to 80 beats per minute
- An athlete's respiration rate will range from 10 to 15 breaths per minute
- Pupils should be equal and constrict with light and dilate with no light

1A. Did you remove the face mask before starting the history? It is recommended that you remove the face mask even though the athlete is breathing with no difficulty. Why? This is a safety measure in case the athlete stops breathing during the assessment. Without the face mask, rescue breathing and CPR is much easier.

During the history, did you ask the athlete about the following?
- headache
- diplopia
- blurred vision
- feeling in legs and arms
- tinnitus
- nausea
- what happened
- what hurts
- retrograde amnesia questions
- post-traumatic amnesia questions
- logic and recall questions
- previous injury to the head or neck

1B. During the observation, did you observe for the following?
- bleeding or fluid from ears, nose, mouth
- bumps, deformities, other signs of trauma
- the athlete's body position
- discoloration, swelling
- skin color
- pupil size

During palpation, did you palpate:
- the neck for bumps, deformities, and point tenderness
- sensory function of the brachial plexus and sacral plexus bilaterally
- motor function of the brachial plexus and sacral plexus bilaterally
- injuries to other parts of the body other than head or neck

1C. Before removing the athlete from the field, did you have the athlete sit up slowly, asking about increased dizziness or headache? Did you use the two-person assistance procedure to get the athlete off the field?

With the athlete on the sideline, did you continue the assessment by:
- having the athlete sit and recheck vitals including pupillary reaction to light
- reasking questions about headache, dizziness, nausea, memory, blurred vision, tinnitus, sensory, and motor functions
- repalpating the neck and checking for range of motion
- check balance by using Romberg's test, sobriety test, and finger to nose test

1D. After completing the assessment, you found that the athlete had a mild headache and sore neck. Did you decide that since the athlete was never unconscious that he could return to the game if he becomes asymptomatic?

 Brachial Plexus Injury

(Refer to pages 557 to 558 in the text)

During the observation of the quarterback's arm, did you observe for:
- swelling, deformity, discoloration, other signs of trauma
- the body position of the athlete and how he was treating his injury
- skin color

2 Brachial Plexus Injury (Con't)

During palpation, did you palpate for:
- swelling, deformity
- point tenderness of the neck and shoulder region
- sensory function of the brachial plexus nerves
- motor function of the brachial plexus nerves

During the special tests, did you:
- check range of motion for the neck and shoulder region
- check strength of the brachial plexus myotomes, particularly the biceps, deltoid, and external rotators
- check grip strength

2A. Did you determine that if the athlete has no related neck or shoulder injury that he could return to the game if strength of the biceps returns to normal?

3 Lumbar Spine Injury

(Refer to Tables 14-4 [page 562] , 14-5 [page 564], and 14-8 [page 574 in the text])

During palpation, did you palpate for:
- swelling, muscle spasms, point tenderness, deformities, other trauma
- bony structures, soft tissue, muscles

3A. During the special test, did you use the straight leg test to determine nerve root involvement or sciatica? Did you use the valsalva test to determine disc injury? Did you check the Achilles tendon reflex?

3B. Did you determine that if the athlete had signs of nerve root involvement or disc injury that referral to a physicians is warranted?

V. Situations

1. Neck Strain - Refer to page 556 and Figures 14-24A to D on text pages 572 to 573 - During the testing procedures, did you have the athlete
- perform forward bending, looking for 80 degrees of flexion
- perform backward bending, looking for 90 degrees of extension
- perform sidebending, looking for 45 degrees of bending
- perform rotation, looking for 90 degrees of rotation

V. Situations (Con't)

Did you have the athlete perform these movements both actively and against manual resistance?

2. Thoracic Spine Injury - Did you palpate the following structures for point tenderness, deformity, muscle spasms, swelling, and temperature during your assessment?
- thoracic spinous processes
- intervertebral ligaments
- intervertebral muscles
- latissimus dorsi

Did you perform the following special tests?
- forward bending and extension
- lateral bending and rotation
- deep breathing
- shoulder flexion, extension, abduction, adduction, horizontal flexion, and extension
- movements of the butterfly stroke

Did you determine that since the swimmer was an adolescent and that the movement associated with the butterfly stroke caused pain that the swimmer may have Scheuermann's disease?

VI. Special Tests

Refer to pages 571 to 578 in the text.

VII. Multiple Choice Answers

1. c	8. d	15. a
2. a	9. c	16. b
3. c	10. d	17. c
4. b	11. b	18. b
5. d	12. a	19. b
6. a	13. b	20. c
7. c	14. c	

Chapter 15 — Throat, Thorax and Visceral Injuries

After completing this chapter you should be able to:

- Locate the important bony and soft tissue structures of the throat, thorax, and viscera

- Recognize specific injuries of the throat, thorax, and viscera

- Describe the life-threatening conditions that can occur spontaneously or as a result of direct trauma to the throat, thorax, and viscera

- Demonstrate an assessment of the throat, thorax, and visceral regions

- Describe the pelvic/abdominal stabilization exercises and abdominal strengthening exercises

I. Anatomy Review

Materials Needed:

SKELETON   ANATOMICAL CHARTS OF THE THROAT, THORAX, AND VISCERAL REGIONS
NONPERMANENT MARKERS

Instructions: *Work with a partner to perform the following:*
- *identify the following anatomical structures on the skeleton or anatomical charts*
- *palpate and draw the anatomical structures on your partner (where appropriate) using the nonpermanent marker.*

Structures of the Throat

-pharynx
-larynx
-trachea
-esophagus
-carotid arteries
-superior thyroid artery

-facial artery
-lingual artery
-subclavian artery
-costocervical artery
-thyrocervical trunk artery
-vertebral artery

Structures of the Thorax

-thoracic cage (sternum, ribs, costal
   cartilage, thoracic vertebrae)
-pleura
-bronchial tubes
-heart
-pectoralis minor
-serratus anterior

-subclavius
-levator scapulae
-trapezius
-rhomboids
-external intercostals
-internal intercostals
-diaphragm

Structures of the Visceral Region

-spleen
-liver
-pancreas
-kidneys
-adrenal glands
-stomach
-small and large intestines
-bladder
-ureter
-appendix
-gallbladder
-sacrum
-ischium
-pubis
-ilium

-aorta
-left and right coronary arteries
-left and right common carotid arteries
-brachial arteries
-intercostal arteries
-renal arteries
-splenic artery
-hepatic artery
-rectus abdominis
-external oblique
-internal oblique
-transverse abdominous
-quadratus lumborum
-inguinal ligament
-linea alba

II. Key Terms

Instructions: *Define the following terms.*

Alveoli
Pulmonary circuit
Systemic circuit
Atria
Ventricles
Vocal cords
Atrioventricular valves
Semilunar valves
Chyme
Peristalsis
Hepatitis
Cirrhosis
Laryngospasm

Flail chest
Runner's nipple
Cyclist's nipple
Gynecomastia
Stitch-in-side
Hyperventilation
Pulmonary contusion
Subcutaneous emphysema
Pneumothorax
Tension pneumothorax
Traumatic asphyxia
Hemothorax
Arrhythmia

Sudden death
Marfan's syndrome
Athletic heart syndrome
Solar plexus punch
Hernia
Peritonitis
Infectious mononucleosis
Kehr's sign
Appendicitis
McBurney's point
Hematuria
Proteinuria

III. Simulations

Instructions: *Perform the following simulated experiences.*

A cyclist was riding over loose gravel on the road when the rear tire skidded sideways causing the rider to fall. During the fall, the rider fell forward onto the handlebars. The rider is complaining of pain on the right lower side of the rib cage. Explain and demonstrate palpations and special testing procedures for this injury.

1A. Palpation reveals point tenderness over the lower right rib cage. There is no deformity or crepitation noted. However, during coughing and deep breaths, the cyclist experiences severe pain in the injured area. Manual lateral compression of the rib cage also increases the intensity of pain. What injury do you suspect and how will you manage this injury?

A football defensive back was making a tackle with his right arm extended. He reports feeling a snapping sensation over his right upper chest wall and complains of an aching fatigue like pain. Explain what factors should be observed in this injury.

2A. Observation reveals swelling and ecchymosis to the anterior right chest wall. Deformity is noted medially to the chest wall. Continue the evaluation with special testing.

2B. Shoulder motion is limited by pain during range of motion, and horizontal adduction and internal rotation are weak. What may be present?

A second baseman fielded a base hit and threw the ball to first base. By accident, the ball struck a base runner going to second base directly on the sternum. The runner immediately collapsed on the base path. You arrived at the scene to find the player in obvious pain and gasping for air. How will you manage this situation? What would indicate the need for EMS?

3A. What underlying serious problems do you need to be concerned about during the treatment of this injury?

A colleague was playing flag football when a sudden back hyperextension injury caused sharp pain in the abdominal region. There is marked tenderness and muscle guarding slightly below and to the right of the umbilicus. No swelling or discoloration is visible, nor is there radiating pain. Explain and demonstrate palpation and stress test.

4A. During the special tests, the individual complains of pain in the abdominal area during back extension and during a modified sit-up activity. What injury do you suspect?

 A 20-year-old football player was struck in the abdomen with a helmet and experienced a sudden onset of abdominal pain in the upper left quadrant. Complete a history and palpate the appropriate structures for this injury.

5A. During the history, the individual states that he is experiencing radiating pain into his upper chest and left shoulder. He feels weak and lightheaded. Blood pressure is 96/72 and his pulse is weak at 96 beats per minute. Palpation reveals point tenderness and rigidity over the upper left quadrant. What injury do you suspect, and what is your immediate first-aid procedure?

IV. Situations

Instructions: *Work with a partner to cooperatively analyze and answer the following situations.*

1. An ice hockey player was checked into the sideboard. The opponent's elbow inadvertently struck the player's anterior neck. The player is now on the ice coughing and having difficulty swallowing. How will you control the situation and manage the injury?

2. A female runner is complaining of breast soreness. After evaluation you have determined that she may need to purchase a sport bra. Discuss the types of sport bras available and the factors that limit motion and irritation to the breasts.

3. After a long layoff, a cross-country runner complains of a stitch in the side during the initial practice. What advice can you provide to this runner to help alleviate the pain that occurs during running?

4. After running wind sprints, the center on the basketball team is having trouble catching her breath. During the history, she reports that she feels numbness in her lips and hands, is somewhat dizzy, and has a dry mouth. What condition do you suspect, and how will you manage this condition?

IV. Situations (Con't)

5. Marfan's syndrome is a disorder most often associated with individuals who have long tubular bones. You have been asked to screen a basketball team for Marfan's syndrome. Please determine the types of screening procedures used to accomplish this task.

6. A running back has received a severe blow to the abdomen. The athlete is experiencing dyspnea. You suspect a solar plexus contusion. How will you manage this injury?

V. Multiple Choice Questions

Instructions: Choose the best answer for each question.

___1. The contraction phase of the heartbeat is known as _____.
   a. diastole   c. aventricular rhythm
   b. systole   d. palpitations

___2. The major respiratory muscle is the _____.
   a. lungs   c. diaphragm
   b. pleura   d. intercostal

___3. Solid organs of the visceral region include all but which of the following:
   a. bladder   c. kidneys
   b. spleen   d. liver

___4. Functions of the _____ can be severely impaired by cirrhosis and hepatitis.
   a. spleen   c. liver
   b. kidneys   d. heart

___5. The _____ secrete the hormones insulin and glucagon, which respectively lower and elevate blood sugar levels.
   a. gallbladder   c. small intestines
   b. pancreas   d. colon

___6. A sharp pain or spasm in the chest wall usually on the _____ during exertion is referred to as a "stitch in the side."
   a. lower left side   c. upper left side
   b. lower right side   d. upper right side

___7. Cyclist's nipples are a result of _____.
   a. constant friction   c. perspiration and windchill
   b. compression   d. perspiration and friction

___8. Gynecomastia can be a result of _____.
   a. increased weight lifting   c. anabolic steroid use
   b. amino acid use   d. over developed pectoralis muscles

___9. During a rupture of the proximal attachment of the pectoralis major muscle, the muscle will _____.
   a. retract toward the axillary fold c. stay in a neutral position
   b. retract into the chest region   d. bleed into the chest cavity

__10. A football player walks off the field leaning toward his right side. Upon evaluation he cannot take a deep breath, and lateral compression test is positive. What injury do you suspect?
a. rectus abdominis strain   c. rib fracture
b. contusion to the sternum   d. pneumothorax

__11. To treat an athlete who is experiencing hyperventilation, you would have the athlete:
a. lie down with the feet elevated
b. have the athlete concentrate on slow inhalations through the nose and exhaling through the mouth
c. have the athlete inhale and exhale through the mouth
d. provide oxygen for the athlete

__12. A baseball pitcher has been struck on the chest with a hard driven baseball. He collapses and goes into respiratory arrest. What injury do you suspect?
a. arrhythmia   c. hypertrophic cardiomyopathy
b. traumatic asphyxia   d. cardiac tamponade

__13. Individuals with Marfan's syndrome normally have _____.
a. enlarged hearts   c. short tubular bones
b. long tubular bones   d. congenital heart failure

__14. _____ should never be placed on open wounds of the abdominal region.
a. sterile water   c. ointments or creams
b. ice   d. absorbent pads

__15. An athlete has received a blow to the abdomen and is experiencing dyspnea. This injury is referred to as a _____.
a. brachial plexus punch   c. celiac plexus punch
b. solar plexus punch   d. contusion

__16. _____ hernias are rare but are more commonly seen in women.
a. congenital   c. direct inguinal
b. indirect inguinal   d. femoral

__17. An athlete who has a hernia may have aching pain in the _____.
a. groin   c. lower back
b. left lower quadrant   d. pubic symphysis

__18. Referred pain down the left shoulder during spleen injury is due to irritation of the diaphragm innervated by the _____.
a. brachial nerve   c. phrenic nerve
b. subclavian nerve   d. thoracic nerve

__19. Rebound pain over the lower right quadrant with referred pain to the lower back may be indicative of _____.
a. appendicitis   c. hernia
b. ruptured bladder   d. spastic colon

__20. McBurney's point is associated with _____.
a. rebound pain with bladder injuries   c. rebound pain with appendicitis
b. injuries to the kidneys   d. injuries to the testicles

VI. Additional Activities

1. Visit a medical facility and ask if you can view x-rays of the thorax and abdominal region.

2. Pick an injury of the thorax or abdominal region, research the injury, and write a paper.

3. Stop by the emergency medical service in your neighborhood and talk with the EMTs and paramedics about internal injuries including heart conditions that they have treated.

Student's Key

I. Anatomy

Refer to Table 15-1 on page 592 in the text.

II. Key Terms

Alveoli — — — — — — — Air sacs at the terminal ends of the bronchial tree where oxygen and carbon dioxide are exchanged between the lungs and surrounding capillaries

Pulmonary circuit — — — Blood vessels that transport unoxygenated blood to the lungs from the right heart ventricle and oxygenated blood from the lungs to the left atrium

Systemic circuit — — — — Blood vessels that transport unoxygenated blood to the right heart atrium and oxygenated blood from the left heart ventricle

Atria — — — — — — — — Two superior chambers of the heart that pump blood into the ventricles

Ventricles — — — — — — Two inferior chambers of the heart that pump blood out of the heart, one to the pulmonary circuit and one to the systemic circuit

Vocal cords — — — — — — Bands of elastic connective tissue encased in mucosal folds that enable the voice to make sound

Atrioventricular valves —— Heart valves that prevent the backflow of blood from the ventricles to the atria

Semilunar valves — — — — Heart valves that prevent the backflow of blood from the pulmonary artery and aorta to the ventricles

Chyme — — — — — — — Paste-like substance into which food is churned in the stomach

Peristalsis — — — — — — Periodic waves of smooth muscle contraction that propel food through the digestive system

Hepatitis — — — — — — — Inflammation of the liver

Cirrhosis — — — — — — — Progressive inflammation of the liver usually caused by alcoholism

II. Key Terms (Con't)

Laryngospasm — — — — — Spasmodic closure of the glottic aperture, leading to shortness of breath, coughing, cyanosis and even loss of consciousness

Flail chest — — — — — — Three or more consecutive ribs on the same side of the chest wall that are fractured in at least two separate locations

Runner's nipple — — — — Nipple irritation due to friction as the shirt rubs over the nipples

Cyclist's nipple — — — — Nipple irritation due to the combined effects of perspiration and windchill producing cold, painful nipples

Gynecomastia — — — — — Excessive development of the male mammary glands

Stitch-in-side — — — — — A sharp pain or spasm in the chest wall, usually on the lower right side, that occurs during exertion

Hyperventilation — — — — Respiratory condition where too much carbon dioxide is exhaled, leading to an inability to catch one's breath

Pulmonary contusion — — Contusion to the lungs due to compressive force

Subcutaneous emphysema – Presence of air or gas in subcutaneous tissue, characterized by a crackling sensation on palpation

Pneumothorax — — — — Condition whereby air is trapped in the pleural space causing a portion of a lung to collapse

Tension pneumothorax —— Condition in which air continuously leaks into the pleural space, causing the mediastinum to displace to the opposite side and compresses the uninjured lung and thoracic aorta

Traumatic asphyxia — — — Condition involving extravasation of blood into the skin and conjunctivae due to sudden increase in venous pressure

Hemothorax — — — — — Condition involving the loss of blood into the pleural cavity, but outside the lung

Arrhythmia — — — — — — Disturbance in heartbeat rhythm

Sudden death — — — — — Nontraumatic, unexpected death occurring instantaneously or within minutes of an abrupt change in an individual's previous clinical state

II. Key Terms (Con't)

Marfan's syndrome — — — Inherited connective tissue disorder affecting many organs, but commonly resulting in the dilation and weakening of the thoracic aorta

Athletic heart syndrome —— Benign condition associated with physiological alterations in the heart

Solar plexus punch — — — A blow to the abdomen that results in an immediate inability to breathe freely

Hernia — — — — — — — Protrusion of abdominal viscera through a weakened portion of the abdominal wall

Peritonitis — — — — — — Inflammation of the peritoneum that lines the abdomen

Infectious mononucleosis — Viral condition caused by the Epstein-Barr virus that attacks the respiratory system and leaves the spleen enlarged and weak

Kehr's sign — — — — — — Referred pain into the left shoulder due to a ruptured spleen

Appendicitis — — — — — Inflammation of the appendix

McBurney's point — — — A site one-third the distance between the ASIS and umbilicus that ,with deep palpation, produces rebound tenderness indicating appendicitis

Hematuria — — — — — — Blood and red blood cells in the urine

Proteinuria — — — — — — Abnormal concentrations of protein in the urine

III. Simulations

1 Rib Fracture

(Refer to text pages 602–604 and Field Strategy 15-2 on text page 603)

During palpation, did you palpate bilaterally for:
- point tenderness
- crepitation
- deformity
- spasm
- rebound pain

Rib Fracture (Con't)

During special tests, did you:
- have the athlete cough and take deep breaths, noting if pain or other symptoms were associated with the injured area?
- apply manual lateral compression to the rib cage, testing for possible rib fracture?
- perform range of motion testing for the trunk, noting increased pain during lateral flexion away from the injured area?

1A. Did you suspect the cyclist may have a rib fracture?
- Did you apply ice to minimize pain and inflammation, immobilize the area, and refer the individual to a physician?

2 **Rupture of the Pectoralis Major Muscle**

(Refer to page 601 in the text)

During observation, did you observe bilaterally for:
- swelling
- eccyhmosis
- deformity
- other signs of trauma

2A. During special tests, did you do the following bilaterally, noting limits in range of motion, muscular weakness, and motions that increase pain?
- active, passive, and resistive range of motion of the shoulder in flexion/extension, abduction/adduction, internal/external rotation, horizontal adduction/abduction
- functional movements

2B. Did you suspect the defensive back ruptured the right pectoralis major muscle?

 Respiratory Distress

The runner is in obvious respiratory distress. During the management of this injury, did you:
- initiate a primary survey
- talk to the athlete to calm them down
- assess breathing and circulation
- take vital signs
- treat for shock

3 **Respiratory Distress (Con't)**

Did you indicate that EMS would be needed if:
 - respirations did not return to normal
 - cardiac irregularities were present

3A. Did you determine that the impact of the ball may have caused:
 - hyperventilation
 - fractured sternum
 - internal complications to the heart or lungs

4 **Rectus Abdominus Muscle Strain**

During special tests, did you have the individual perform the following, noting limits in range motion, weakness, and increased pain?
 - active, passive, and resistive trunk flexion/extension, lateral flexion, and rotation
 - modified sit-ups

4A. Because pain increases with active contraction of the abdominal muscles during a modified sit-up, did you suspect this injury was a strain to the rectus abdominus or obliques?

5 **Ruptured Spleen**

Refer to Table 15-5 on page 611 and Field Strategies 15-3, 15-4 and 15-5, and 15-6 on text pages 611, 614, 616, and 620, respectively.

During the history, did you:
 - ask where, when, and how questions
 - ask about the type of pain the athlete is experiencing
 - ask if the athlete was experiencing any dizziness, nausea, weakness, numbness, or other unusual feelings

Did you check blood pressure and pulse rate?

Did you palpate the upper left quadrant for:
 - point tenderness
 - swelling
 - deformity
 - rebound pain
 - spasms and rigidity

Did you palpate the remaining abdomen?

5A. Did you suspect the football player may have ruptured the spleen? Did your treatment protocol include treating for shock and immediately summoning EMS?

IV. Situations

l. Anterior Throat Trauma - (Refer to Field Strategy 15-1 on page 599 in the text) - To care for the injured hockey player, did you reassure the individual and attempt to place the chin in a forward position to straighten the airway? Did you make note that if breathing does not return to normal within a few minutes EMS should be summoned?

2. Sport Bra Selection - (Refer to Chapter 6, Protective Equipment, in the text, on pages 196–197 and 199.)

3. Stitch in the Side - To alleviate the pain, the runner can:
- forcibly exhale through pursed lips
- breathe deeply and regularly
- lean away from the affected side
- stretch the arm on the affected side over the head as high as possible

4. Hyperventilation - Did you suspect the basketball player is experiencing hyperventilation? Did your management plan include:
- calm the player down
- have the player concentrate on slow inhalations through the nose and exhaling through the mouth to slow breathing
- breathe into a paper bag

5. Marfan's Syndrome Screening - (Refer to pages 606 - 607 and Table 15-4 on text page 60) - Did you include the following screening procedures for Marfan's syndrome?
- height and arm span measurements
- past history of rheumatic fever, hypertension, cardiac problems, or chronic disease
- symptoms of syncope, near syncope, palpitations, low exercise tolerance, chest discomfort on exertion, or dyspnea
- family history of syncope, hypertension, premature coronary disease, or sudden death
- measurements of blood pressure and pulse, auscultation of the heart for cardiac rhythm, murmurs, and abnormal heart sounds, and palpation of peripheral pulses

IV. Situations (Con't)

6. Solar Plexus Contusion - Did you manage the solar plexus contusion by:
- assessing airway for obstruction
- removing any mouthguard or dental apparatus
- loosening restrictive clothing and/or equipment around the abdomen
- having the individual flex his knees toward his chest
- summoning EMS if breathing does not return to normal within a few minutes

V. Multiple Choice Answers

1. b	8. c	15. b
2. c	9. a	16. d
3. a	10. c	17. a
4. c	11. b	18. c
5. b	12. d	19. a
6. b	13. b	20. c
7. c	14. c	

Chapter 16 — Conditions Related to the Reproductive System

After completing this chapter you should be able to:

- List the primary and accessory organs in the female and male reproductive system

- Explain the signs and symptoms of common injuries to the female and male genitalia

- Describe management of injuries to the female and male genitalia

- Indicate the mode of transmission, signs and symptoms, and current treatment of sexually transmitted diseases.

- Identify the various menstrual irregularities and the implications they may have on sport participation

- Describe how sport performance may be affected by the use of oral contraceptives and IUDs

- Specify indications and contraindications for sport participation during pregnancy

I. Anatomy Review

Materials Needed:
SKELETON   ANATOMICAL CHARTS

Instructions: *Identify the following anatomical structures on the skeleton or anatomical charts and explain the function of each structure.*

Anatomy of the Genitalia

-ovaries

-testes

-fallopian tubes

-uterus

-vagina

-vulva

-epididymis

-ductus deferens

-seminal vesicles

-prostate gland

-bulbourethral gland

-scrotum

-penis

-pelvic girdle

II. Key Terms

Instructions: *Define the following key terms.*

Primary sex organs   Androgens   Retroviruses
Accessory sex organs   Hydrocele   Dysmenorrhea
Steroids   Varicocele   Oligomenorrhea
Menses   Hematocele   Amenorrhea
Estrogens   Pruritus   Osteopenia
Progesterone

III. Simulations

Instructions: *Perform the following experiences.*

 A soccer player was struck in the groin by a knee. He was not wearing a protective cup and immediately fell to the ground. What possible conditions can occur as a result of direct trauma to the male genitalia?

1A. The soccer player has sustained injury to the testicles and they are in spasm. Explain and demonstrate how to manage the condition. What signs and symptoms would indicate referral to a physician is necessary?

 A basketball player is complaining of painful urination and has open sores on the penis. What might you suspect, and how will you address your concerns with the athlete? What advice will you provide to the athlete?

2A. The basketball player has been diagnosed with a sexually transmitted disease. He has been warned to avoid sexual contact with anyone until his next appointment with the physician. What can be done in the work environment to prevent the spread of sexually transmitted diseases?

 After watching a softball player for the past 3 weeks, you suspect she may have hepatitis. She appears lethargic, easily tires, and has notable signs of yellowing in the whites of her eyes. What clues in the history would confirm your suspicions?

3A. After referring the softball player to the physician, your hunch was confirmed, and she was diagnosed with hepatitis. What type of treatment will the player need to follow?

IV. Situations

Instructions: *Work with a partner to cooperatively analyze and answer the following situations.*

l. A cyclist is complaining of transient paresthesia of his penis when riding for long periods of time. What condition might you suspect? What anatomical structure is involved, and what preventative measures can prevent this condition from recurring?

2. A baseball team has been struck with an outbreak of tinea cruris. You have been asked to educate the team on prevention and then discuss treatment for this condition.

3. A lean 16-year-old distance runner has reported she has not had a menstrual period in 3 months and is concerned that she may be pregnant. What other menstrual irregularities could account for this absence of menses?

4. A female gymnast is experiencing dysmenorrhea and is having difficulty getting through practice because of the discomfort. Indicate how you would treat this woman for this condition.

5. A female athlete wants to begin taking oral contraceptives for birth control reasons. What implications may these oral contraceptives have on her performance, and what adverse effects might she experience? Please discuss these with the athlete.

6. A recreational runner has asked for information concerning running and exercise during pregnancy. What advice can you provide?

V. Multiple Choice Questions

Instructions: Choose the best answer for each question.

___l.   The epididymis, prostate gland, and seminal vesicles are all _____.
a. female accessory sex organs   c. primary sex organs
b. male accessory sex organs   d. female reproductive organs

___2.   The female reproductive organs are protected by the _____ and are seldom injured during sport participation.
a. pelvic girdle   c. rectus femoris
b. iliac crest   d. sacroiliac joint structures

___3.   _____ help(s) regulate the menstrual cycle and influence the development of female physical sex characteristics.
a. testosterone   c. estrogens
b. progesterone   d. steroids

___4.   Transient paresthesia of the penis during cycling can be decreased by:
a. adjusting the pedals   c. adjusting the handlebar height
b. adjusting the saddle position   d. wearing padded cycling shorts

___5. To relieve muscle spasms of the testicles, you can _____.
   a. apply superficial heat
   b. have the athlete apply direct pressure to the area
   c. place the athlete on his back and flex his knees toward his chest
   d. have the athlete perform static trunk and hip hyperextension

___6. Most injuries to the vulva involve _____.
   a. a forced perineal stretching during sudden leg abduction
   b. a forced perineal stretching during sudden leg extension
   c. infection
   d. past medical history of injury

___7. Tinea cruris is a _____ infection involving the genitalia.
   a. bacterial   c. chemical
   b. viral   d. fungal

___8. Tinea cruris grows optimally in all but which of the following?
   a. dark environment   c. dry environment
   b. warm environment   d. moist environment

___9. "Chub rub" is a term used to describe _____.
   a. intertrigo of the axillary area   c. intertrigo of the thighs
   b. tinea cruris   d. contact dermatitis

__10. _____ is a yeast infection found in women.
   a. trichomoniasis   c. chlamydia
   b. gonorrhea   d. candidiasis

__11. Hepatitis primarily attacks the _____, impairing function.
   a. liver   c. kidneys
   b. lungs   d. reproductive organs

__12. The vaccine immunoglobulin ___can prevent hepatitis B and should be administered to individuals who are at risk for coming in contact with the virus.
   a. IG   c. IGB
   b. IGC   d. GI

__13. The HIV virus attacks and destroys several cells in the body's immune system, particularly the _____ known as the helper T-cell.
   a. monocyte   c. lymphocyte
   b. erythrocyte   d. chondrocyte

__14. According to the American Academy of Pediatrics, athletes with HIV should be allowed to participate in _____.
   a. all sports   c. noncollision sports
   b. noncontact sports   d. no sports

__15. ____ is the best protection for an athletic trainer to use to keep from getting AIDS.
   a. use of birth control methods during intercourse
   b. using latex gloves when dealing with blood and bodily fluids
   c. getting the HBV vaccination
   d. using biohazardous waste disposal containers

___16. Menorrhagia can lead to ____ depletion which affects athletic performance.
- a. electrolyte
- b. calcium
- c. amino acid
- d. iron

___17. A female athlete has stopped having her menstrual cycle for 6 months. This condition is considered to be _____.
- a. secondary amenorrhea
- b. primary amenorrhea
- c. osteopenia
- d. dysmenorrhea

___18. Amenorrhea and decreased estrogen predispose women to _____, leading to increased _____.
- a. increased bone density, stress fractures
- b. decreased bone density, stress fractures
- c. decreased bone density, premenstrual syndrome
- d. premenstrual syndrome, stress fractures

___19. Postural adaptations during pregnancy can lead to _____, which increases back pain during pregnancy.
- a. spinal stenosis
- b. scoliosis
- c. lordosis
- d. spondylolysis

___20. _____ movements should be avoided while performing aerobic dance exercises during pregnancy.
- a. static
- b. ballistic
- c. stepping
- d. stretching

VI. Additional Activities

1. Visit the local health department and ask for more information concerning sexually transmitted diseases and AIDS.

2. Trace the female and male reproductive system and determine what conditions and/or injuries may occur to each area.

I. Anatomy

Refer to Figures 16-1 and 16-2 on page 628 in the text.

II. Key Terms

Primary sex organs — — — Reproductive organs responsible for producing gametes (ovum and sperm)

Accessory sex organs — — Organs that transport, protect, and nourish gametes

Steroids — — — — — — A large family of chemical substances including endocrine secretions and hormones

Menses — — — — — — Phase in the menstrual cycle when the thickened vascular walls of the uterus, the unfertilized ova, and blood from damaged vessels are lost during the menstrual flow

Estrogens — — — — — A class of hormones that produce female secondary sex characteristics and affect the menstrual cycle

Progesterone — — — — — Hormone responsible for thickening the uterine lining in preparation for the fertilized ovum

Androgens — — — — — A class of hormones that promote development of male genitals and secondary sex characteristics and influence sexual motivation

Hydrocele — — — — — Swelling in the tunica vaginalis of the testes

Varicocele — — — — — Abnormal dilation of the veins of the spermatic cord leading to engorgement of blood into the spermatic cord veins during a standing position

Hematocele — — — — — A rapid accumulation of blood and fluid in the scrotum around the testicle and cord

Pruritus — — — — — — Intense itching

Retroviruses — — — — — Any virus of the family Retroviridae known to reverse the usual order of reproduction within the cells they infect

Dysmenorrhea — — — — Difficult or painful menstruation; menstrual cramps

II. Key Terms (Con't)

Oligomenorrhea — — — — Infrequent menstrual cycles

Amenorrhea — — — — — Absence or abnormal cessation of menstruation

Osteopenia — — — — — — Decreased calcification or density of bone

III. Simulations

 Testicular Spasm

Did you determine that the following conditions could result from direct trauma to the male genitalia?
- contusion to the testes or penis
- scrotal hemorrhage
- hydrocele
- hematocele
- tunica vaginitis

1A. In your management plan for the injury, did you:
- instruct the individual to bring his knees to his chest to relieve the spasms
- apply cold compresses to reduce swelling and hemorrhage
- treat for shock if needed
- encourage the individual to do periodic self assessment

Did you conclude that the following signs and symptoms would indicate referral to a physician?
- swelling of testicles
- severe discoloration
- increase pain and discomfort

 Sexually Transmitted Disease

(Refer to Table 16-1 on pages 635–637 and Field Strategy 16-2 on text page 640)

Did you suspect a sexually transmitted disease such as herpes or gonorrhea? Did you approach the individual with a caring and sensitive attitude, suggesting the individual seek medical attention as soon as possible and refrain from any sexual contact until after the appointment?

2A. Did you suggest following OSHA standards governing exposure to blood-borne pathogens to prevent the spread of these diseases in the work environment?

During the history, did you identify the following factors to suggest the individual may have hepatitis?
- yellowing of eyes
- mild flu-like symptoms
- poor appetite
- nausea
- dizziness
- general muscle aches
- fatigue and headaches
- abdominal pain

3A. Did you include the following as part of the treatment protocol for hepatitis?
- bed rest
- plenty of fluids

IV. Situations

l. Biker's Penis - Did you determine that the cyclist was experiencing biker's penis as a result of pressure to the pudendal nerve? Did you suggest the following measures to prevent this condition from recurring:
- adjusting the height and tilt of the saddle
- adjusting the number of cycling bouts
- standing up on the pedals periodically to relieve the pressure on the affected nerve

2. Tinea Cruris - (Refer to Field Strategy 16-l on text page 634) - Did your preventive measures include:
- proper drying after showers
- wearing cotton briefs and shorts
- wearing nonrestrictive shorts and briefs
- keeping the area dry with powders

Did your treatment protocol include:
- application of antifungal agents such as Micatin, Lotrimin, Mycelex, or Tinactin twice daily for at least 1 month
- keeping the area clean and dry
- wearing absorbent clothing such as those made from cotton
- if the condition does not clear, refer to a physician

3. Menstrual Irregularities - Other than pregnancy, did you suggest that the distance runner could also be experiencing secondary amenorrhea and should be seen by a physician to rule out pregnancy?

4. Dysmenorrhea - Did you suggest the following for treating the dysmenorrhea?
- over-the-counter medications such as Midol, Advil, or Ibuprofen to relieve the pain and cramping
- eating a diet high in fiber and fluid and low in salt to decrease the risk of dysmenorrhea

5. Oral Contraceptives - **(Refer to text pages 643–644)** - Did you suggest that oral contraceptives can increase the risk for certain conditions but low dose oral contraceptives and regular exercise can offset many of the risks providing a safe effective birth control method for active women.

6. Exercise During Pregnancy - **(Refer to Field Strategy 16-3 on page 646 and Table 16-6 on text page 647)** - Did you determine that exercise problems of pregnant women include:
- poor balance
- overheating and dehydration
- leg, hip, or abdominal pain
- avoiding weight-loading activities such as volleyball, basketball, or horseback riding
- avoiding ballistic activity and doing no impact aerobics
- weight training with lightweight and high repetitions
- decreasing running distance and intensity as pregnancy progresses
- consult a physician before starting or continuing any exercise program

V. Multiple Choice Answers

1. b	8. c	15. b
2. a	9. c	16. d
3. c	10. d	17. a
4. b	11. a	18. b
5. c	12. c	19. c
6. a	13. c	20. b
7. d	14. a	

Chapter 17 — Other Health Conditions Related to Sports

After completing this chapter you should be able to:

- Identify what impact environmental conditions, such as altitude and poor air quality, have on sport participation

- Describe the signs, symptoms, and management of common respiratory tract infections

- Describe the signs, symptoms, and management of common disorders of the gastrointestinal tract

- Explain the physiological factors involved in diabetes and differentiate the management of diabetic coma from insulin shock

- Identify common contagious viral diseases

- Describe the signs and management of an individual experiencing an epileptic seizure

- List common substances abused by athletes and the impact on the individual's health and sport performance

- Describe the various eating disorders and explain guidelines for safe weight loss and weight gain

I. Key Terms

Instructions: *Define the following terms.*

Hypoxia
Rhinitis
Rhinorrhea
Malaise
Sinusitis
Pharyngitis
Influenza
Hay fever
Bronchitis
Infectious mononucleosis
Asthma

Bronchospasm
Gastroenteritis
Diarrhea
Constipation
Hemorrhoids
Diabetes
Hyperglycemia
Hypoglycemia
Epilepsy
Clonic state

Tonic state
Hypertension
Anemia
Sickle cell anemia
Infarcts
Therapeutic drugs
Antipyretic
Neoplasm
Bulimia
Anorexia nervosa

II. Simulations

Instructions: *Perform the following simulated experiences.*

 A volleyball player has suddenly developed a headache, general body aches, and is slightly chilled. To determine if the individual is developing the flu, what other questions would you ask, and what observations might confirm your suspicions? Demonstrate how to determine if this individual has a fever.

1A. After doing a more thorough history and observation, you have determined that the volleyball player may indeed be experiencing flu-like symptoms. How would you manage this condition?

 A soccer player has been running up and down the field during full contact practice. After a few minutes, the individual begins to experience tightness in the chest, shortness of breath, and wheezing. Complete a history on this sport participant.

2A. You have discovered that the individual has a past history of these episodes and is an asthmatic. What condition is occurring, and what is your immediate treatment protocol?

 A diabetic basketball player is halfway through a practice session when suddenly the player feels weak and faint. Explain and demonstrate how to determine if this player is experiencing insulin shock.

3A. Observations and palpations reveal the individual has pale, cold, and clammy skin and shallow respirations. The individual is perspiring profusely. Explain and demonstrate how to manage this condition.

 A middle-aged female endurance runner is complaining of chronic fatigue and malaise, particularly when running. She appears somewhat pale and tired, but otherwise is fine. Complete a medical history of the condition.

4A. During the history, the runner reports that she tends to have a heavy menstrual flow and does not eat meat or take iron supplements. What condition might you suspect, and how will you manage this runner?

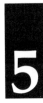

A 16-year-old football player returned from summer vacation 30 pounds heavier and able to bench press 50 additional pounds. Although he reported that he was on an aggressive weight training program over the summer, you question how these gains were made in such a short period of time. How would you further question this athlete about his increased strength gains?

5A. After talking with the football player you suspect he has been taking some sort of tissue-enhancing drug during his summer weight training program. Discuss with the athlete the implications these drugs may have on his health and performance. What follow-up discussions might you have with him?

A baseball player reports to you complaining of inner gum pain. Please perform an observation for this complaint.

6A. You observed white patches on the gums and stained teeth. When asked if the baseball athlete uses smokeless tobacco, he answers yes. Discuss the health implications of smoke-less tobacco with this athlete.

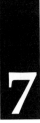

There are rumors that a swimmer was seen eating a large amount of food and then disappeared to the restroom to vomit. After returning from the restroom, her eyes appear bloodshot and she looks pale. There is also rumor that she uses diuretics; however, weight appears normal. What other signs and symptoms would you look for in this athlete that might indicate an eating disorder? Do these rumors need to be addressed? If yes, how will you address them?

7A. After addressing these issues with the athlete, she denies having a dysfunctional eating disorder. What is your next plan of action?

7B. To prevent other swimmers from dysfunctional eating behavior, you have been asked to talk with the team about the proper weight loss that will not affect their performance. Discuss the type of information you would provide in your meeting with the swimmers.

III. Situations

Instructions: *Work with a partner to cooperatively analyze and answer the following situations.*

l. A 37-year-old male with asthma is seeking advice about how to improve his cardiovascular endurance. What activities might you recommend and what guidelines should be followed in developing the exercise program?

2. It is in the spring of the year, and the pollen index is high. A hurdler on the track team reports to practice with itchy and watery eyes. During the warm-up running session, the individual experiences difficulty in breathing and becomes congested. What condition do you suspect, and how would you manage this condition?

3. A male distance runner has reported the consistent need to stop and have a bowel movement while training. Is this normal for runners? What can be done about it?

4. A football player has been having bouts of diarrhea. What type of precautionary measures must be taken if this athlete is going to participate?

5. A tennis player has been diagnosed as a diabetic. The diabetes does not preclude activity or competition. Discuss how to prevent hypoglycemia episodes during exercise.

6. During warm-up, a softball player suddenly gets a glassy stare on the face, begins to smack the lips, and walks aimlessly around the field as if intoxicated. You have determined that the athlete has not been drinking or taking any medications. What condition might this individual have, and how will you manage this situation?

7. A college wrestler wants to lose weight quickly. You have heard that he may be taking diuretics to aid him in his weight loss. Discuss the problems associated with health and performance from taking diuretics as weight loss agents.

8. An athlete has suffered a severe knee injury. You have applied ice, compression, and elevation. You would like to recommend the individual take something for the pain. What type of over-the-counter medication might you recommend and why?

9. During twice a day practices in August, a good number of football players decided to go out and drink during a day off. The next day in practice there were bouts of muscle cramping, and the athletes were just not as sharp with their motor skills as in previous practices. What may have contributed to the decreases in motor skill performance and increased muscle cramping and why?

10. The track and field team is competing in 3 weeks at nationals in Denver, Colorado. Because of the high altitude, what can be done to reduce the impact of altitude on the athletes' performance?

IV. Multiple Choice Questions

Instructions: Choose the best answer for each question.

___1.   The _____ as one ascends above sea level making it more difficult to perform aerobic activity.
a. percentage of oxygen decreases   c. the density of air decreases
b. percentage of carbon dioxide increases   d. the density of air increases

___2.   Diets _____ and _____ in salt can lessen the effects of altitude.
a. high in carbohydrates and low   c. high in protein and low
b. low in carbohydrates and low   d. low in fats and high

___3.   _____ is the single most important factor in the prevention of altitude sickness and hyperthermia.
a. diet   c. acclimatization
b. fluid replenishment   d. clothing

___4.   The _____ sinuses are most commonly involved with sinusitis.
a. sphenoid   c. ethmoid and frontal
b. maxillary and frontal   d. frontal

___5.   The Epstein-Barr virus in the Herpes family is the organism known to cause ____.
a. bronchitis   c. allergic rhinitis
b. influenza   d. infectious mononucleosis

___6.   The single most determining factor used to return a player to participation after having mononucleosis is _____.
a. normal liver function   c. return of energy
b. no signs of sore throat   d. functional ability

___7.   Exercise-induced asthma usually develops shortly after _____ of strenuous exercise.
a. cessation   c. 6 to 8 minutes
b. an hour   d. intermittent period

___8.   Individuals suffering from all but which of the following may be at increased risk for exercise-induced asthma.
a. hyperventilation   c. allergies
b. sinus disease   d. mononucleosis

___9.   A major concern of the athletic trainer when an athlete is suffering from diarrhea is:
a. dehydration leading to heat illness   c. painful abdominal cramps
b. fatigue leading to mononucleosis   d. dizziness and headache

___10.   If a conscious person is suffering from hypoglycemia, give the person ____.
a. gatorade   c. a source of sugar
b. water   d. a source of protein

___11.   The best way to treat an athlete who is having a tonic-clonic seizure is to ____.
a. hold and constrain the athlete
b. place a spoon in the athlete's mouth to prevent the athlete from biting the tongue
c. apply ice to the neck of the athlete
d. remove nearby objects to protect the athlete and allow the athlete to continue through the seizure

___12. Dinabol, Anavar, and Danocrin are all examples of _____.
   a. human growth hormone   c. amphetamines
   b. beta blockers   d. anabolic steroids

___13. In sports participation, anemia contributes to all of the following except _____.
   a. increase in aerobic capacity   c. decrease in aerobic threshold
   b. decrease in aerobic capacity   d. decrease exercise time to exhaustion

___14. In the female athlete, iron-deficiency anemia is mostly seen in _____.
   a. basketball players
   b. those who maintain percent body fat
   c. those who maintain low percent body fat
   d. African-American athletes

___15. Sickle cell anemia is most commonly seen in _____.
   a. African-Americans   c. male athletes
   b. female athletes   d. Asian-Americans

___16. Drugs sold over the counter generally have a dosage of no more than _____.
   a. 500 mg   c. 200 mg
   b. 100 mg   d. 250 mg

___17. NSAIDS are used for all but which of the following?
   a. reduce inflammation   c. reduce pain
   b. reduce fever   d. produce general anesthesia

___18. All but which of the following is used to build muscle mass?
   a. clenbuterol   c. anabolic steroids
   b. corticosteroid   d. human growth hormone

___19. Because of its _____, aspirin should never be administered during the acute phase of an injury.
   a. antipyretic factor   c. anticoagulant factor
   b. antitussive factor   d. anti-inflammation factor

___20. Alcohol is a _____.
   a. central nervous system stimulant   c. ergogenic aid
   b. central nervous system depressant   d. antitussive agent

V. Additional Activities

1. **Visit a pharmacist and ask him to explain the legal ramifications associated with the dispensing of both prescription and over-the-counter medications.**

2. **Visit the pharmacy section of a grocery store and examine all the various types of medications that might be used in treating athletic injuries and illnesses.**

3. **Visit with a counselor who has expertise in alcohol, drug, or food addictions and discuss these various addiction problems.**

4. **Visit an open self-help group meeting such as Alcoholics Anomynous, Overeaters Anomynous, or Narcotics Anomynous.**

I. Key Terms

Hypoxia — — — — — — — Reduction of oxygen supply to tissue despite adequate blood flow

Rhinitis — — — — — — — Inflammation of the nasal membranes with excessive mucus production, resulting in nasal congestion and postnasal drip

Rhinorrhea — — — — — — Clear nasal discharge

Malaise — — — — — — — General discomfort; feeling out-of-sorts

Sinusitis — — — — — — — Inflammation of the paranasal sinuses

Pharyngitis — — — — — — Viral, bacterial, or fungal infection of the pharynx, leading to a sore throat

Influenza — — — — — — Acute infectious respiratory tract condition characterized by malaise, headache, dry cough, and general muscle aches

Hay fever — — — — — — Seasonal allergic rhinitis caused by airborne pollens and/or fungus spores

Bronchitis — — — — — — Inflammation of the mucosal lining of the tracheobronchial tree characterized by bronchial swelling, mucus secretions, and dysfunction of the cilia

Infectious mononucleosis — Acute viral disease caused by the Epstein-Barr virus manifested by malaise and fatigue

Asthma — — — — — — — Disease of the lungs characterized by constriction of the bronchial muscles, increased bronchial secretions, and mucosa swelling, all leading to airway narrowing and inadequate airflow during respiration

Bronchospasm — — — — — Contraction of the smooth muscles of the bronchial tubes causing narrowing of the airway

Gastroenteritis — — — — Inflammation of the mucous membrane of the stomach or small intestine

I. Key Terms (Con't)

Diarrhea — — — — — — Loose or watery stool, resulting when food residue rushes through the large intestine before there is sufficient time to absorb the remaining water

Constipation — — — — — Infrequent or incomplete bowel movements

Hemorrhoids — — — — — Dilations of the venous plexus surrounding the rectal and anal area that can become exposed if they protrude internally or externally

Diabetes — — — — — — Metabolic disorder characterized by near or absolute lack of the hormone insulin, or insulin resistance, or both

Hyperglycemia — — — — Abnormally high levels of glucose in the circulating blood that can lead to diabetic coma

Hypoglycemia — — — — Abnormally low levels of glucose in the circulating blood that can lead to insulin shock

Epilepsy — — — — — — Disorder of the brain characterized by recurrent episodes of sudden, excessive discharges of electrical activity in the brain

Clonic state — — — — — Movement marked by repetitive muscle contractions and relaxation in rapid succession

Tonic state — — — — — — Steady rigid muscle contractions with no relaxation

Hypertension — — — — — Sustained elevated blood pressure above the norms of 140 mm Hg systolic or 90 mm Hg diastolic

Anemia — — — — — — Abnormal reduction in red blood cell volume or hemoglobin concentration

Sickle cell anemia — — — Abnormalities in hemoglobin structure, resulting in a characteristic sickle- or crescent-shaped red blood cell that is fragile and unable to transport oxygen

Infarcts — — — — — — Clumping together of cells that block small blood vessels, leading to vascular occlusion, ischemia, and necrosis in organs

Therapeutic drugs — — — Prescribed or over-the-counter medications used to treat an injury or illness

I. Key Terms (Con't)

Antipyretic — — — — — — Medication used to bring a fever down

Neoplasm — — — — — — Mass of tissue that grows more rapidly than normal and may be either benign or malignant

Bulimia — — — — — — — Personality disorder manifested by episodic bouts of binging large amounts of food followed by purging and feelings of guilt, self-disgust, and depression

Anorexia nervosa — — — Personality disorder manifested by extreme aversion toward food resulting in extreme weight loss, amenorrhea, and other physical disorders

II. Simulations

 Flu and Common Cold

The volleyball player had a headache and body aches. Did you ask if the player had or was experiencing:
- chills
- malaise
- general muscle soreness
- a hacking cough
- sore throat

Did you observe for:
- watery eyes
- fatigue
- pale skin

Did you measure the body temperature by using an oral thermometer?
Is this the most accurate way to measure core temperature?

1A. Did your management include:
- rest
- plenty of fluids
- cough medication
- NSAIDS
- physician referral

During the history, did you:
- determine if the athlete needed emergency medical attention by checking the athlete's vital signs
- ask if the athlete had ever experienced these symptoms before
- ask if the athlete had allergies
- ask if the athlete had asthma
- ask if the athlete had been sick recently with an upper respiratory infection

2A. Did you suspect the soccer player may be experiencing exercise-induced asthma?

Did your management plan include:
- a physician referral
- making sure the player adheres to inhalers that the physician may prescribe
- making sure the player has a progressive warm-up prior to exercise and a cool-down period postexercise

(Refer to Field Strategy 17-2 on text page 656 for exercise strategies for individuals with asthma)

3   **Diabetic Athlete...Insulin Shock**

Did you observe for:
- signs of dizziness
- aggressive behavior
- intense hunger
- pale, cold, clammy skin
- profuse sweating
- fainting

Did you palpate for:
- skin temperature
- vital signs

3A. Did your management plan include:
- getting sugar into the individual quickly by placing sugar under the tongue
- physician referral

(Refer to Field Strategies 17-4 on text page 661 and 17-5 on text page 662)

4 Anemia

Did you ask:
  - if the individual has been sick
  - if the individual has eaten that day and what was eaten
  - if she is currently menstruating and how heavy is the flow
  - if she is taking any iron supplements

4A. Did you suspect iron-deficiency anemia in the distance runner based on her age, distance running, and heavy menstrual flow?

Did your management plan include referral to a physician to rule out other underlying conditions?

5 Steroids

Did your questions include:
  - what type of diet the individual was on during the weight training program
  - what type of weight training program he was involved with
  - if the individual was experiencing any mood swings, depression, or violent behavior
  (Refer to Table 17-5 on text page 671)

5A. Did you approach the athlete in a nonthreatening manner, showing care and concern? Did you educate the athlete about the negative effects associated with steroid and other tissue-enhancing drug use? Did you suggest the athlete visit with a physician or counselor?

 6 Smokeless Tobacco Use

Did you observe:
  - periodontal bone loss
  - tooth loss
  - gum irritation
  - white patches on the gums
  - stained teeth

6A. During the discussion about health implications of smokeless tobacco use, did you include:
  - bad breath
  - decreased taste perception
  - periodontal bone loss
  - tooth loss
  - nicotine addiction
  - oral infections and cancer

Did you include the following signs and symptoms during their evaluation?
- depression
- low self-esteem
- gastrointestinal irritation
- irregular menses
- Russell's sign
- chipmunk face

(Refer to Tables 17-9 on text page 677 and 17-10 on text page 679)

Did you conclude that the rumors need to be addressed and that they should approach the individual in a nonthreatening manner? Did the discussion include:
- a caring and concerned attitude
- short- and long-term health effects and the effects on sport performance
- encourage the individual to seek professional counseling
- physician referral

7A. Did your plan of action include:
- continued support for the individual
- observation of the individual
- monitoring vital signs and other health-related measures
- continued encouragement to seek counseling

*You must remember not to be an enabler for the bulimic athlete.

7B. Refer to Tables 17-9 on text page 677; 17-10 on text page 679; 17-11 on text page 680; and Field Strategy 17-7 on text page 670.

III. Situations

1. Asthma and Exercise - Did your exercise protocol include:
- consultation with a physician
- prescription medication
- progressive warm-up and cool-down
- exercising in a warm, humid environment
- avoiding exposure to air pollutants and allergens

(Refer to Field Strategy 17-2 on page 656 in the text)

2. Allergens - Did you suspect the hurdler had allergies? Did your management plan include:
- reducing exposure to the allergen or irritant
- suppressive medication to alleviate symptoms
- hypersensitization to reduce responsiveness to unavoidable allergens

III. Situations (Con't)

3. Irregular Bowl Function - Did you determine that irregular bowl function is not uncommon? Did you suggest the following for treatment of this condition?
- eating a high-fiber diet
- an increase in daily exercise and fluid intake
- over-the-counter medication as recommended by a physician
- if the condition continues, referral to a physician is needed

(Refer to Table 17-1 on text page 657)

4. Diarrhea - Did you include the following precautionary measures for the football player to participate?
- eating a low-fiber diet 24 to 36 hours prior to competition
- taking advantage of the morning gastrocolic reflex
- improving hydration
- taking either Pepto-Bismol, Imodium, or Lomotil for short durations

5. Hypoglycemia Prevention - Did you include the following to prevent hypoglycemia in the tennis player?
- eat a meal 1 to 3 hours prior to activity
- exercise each day at the same time
- administer insulin more than 1 hour prior to activity
- measure blood glucose levels prior to activity
- consume additional carbohydrate foods every 30 to 45 minutes during activity
- drink plenty of fluids

(Refer to Field Strategy 17-5 on text page 662)

6. Complex Partial Seizure - Did you determine that the softball player might be experiencing a complex partial seizure? Did your management plan include:
- looking for a medic alert tag on the individual
- not restricting the individual but helping the person into a supine position
- clear others from around the individual
- refer to physician

(Refer to Field Strategy 17-6 on text page 664)

7. Diuretics - Did you discuss the following adverse affects of using diuretics with the wrestler?
- lower plasma and blood levels
- depletion of glycogen stores, which means decreased energy
- increased electrolyte loss
- impairment of body temperature regulation which increases heat illness
- lower aerobic capacity
- reduction of muscular strength and work performance

III. Situations (Con't)

8. Pain Medication - Did you determine that as long as the individual is not allergic to acetaminophen or ibuprofen, he/she could take these over-the-counter medications safely? The individual should not be given aspirin because it prevents the clotting of blood for up to 7 days. If in doubt about the type of medication to suggest, a physician should be consulted. (Refer to Table 17-4 on pages 667–668 in the text)

9. Alcohol - Did you determine that the following could have been related to the decreased motor skill performance and muscle cramping after a night of drinking?
- alcohol acts as a dehydrant which could lead to muscle cramping
- alcohol can negatively affect alertness, reaction time, judgment, hand-eye coordination, accuracy, and balance up to 48 hours after drinking
(Refer to Table 17-6 on page 673 in the text)

10. Altitude and Performance - Did you suggest that the following can decrease the effects of high altitude on the track and field team?
- arrive 3 days prior to competition
- get plenty of rest
- drink plenty of fluids
- eat a diet high in carbohydrates

IV. Multiple Choice Answers

1. c	8. d	15. a
2. a	9. a	16. c
3. c	10. c	17. d
4. c	11. d	18. b
5. d	12. d	19. c
6. a	13. a	20. b
7. c	14. c	